"If you, or someone you [love ...] liver disease, then this book could [be a] lifesaver. It [offers] not only the most invaluable scientific information and knowledge on the subject, but the wisdom of experience, from one of the foremost hepatologists in the world."

—Deepak Chopra, M.D., F.A.C.P., founder and CEO of the Chopra Center for Well Being, and author of *Perfect Health* and *Ageless Body, Timeless Mind*

Did you know . . .

• The liver has the remarkable ability to regenerate itself? Persons with healthy livers can donate part of their liver to another, and the liver will grow to full size in both people within a few months.

• Itchy and easily bruising skin could be signs of liver disease?

• Roughly 4 million Americans have chronic hepatitis C infection and many do not know it? It has been dubbed "the silent epidemic."

• Simply eating a steak could cause disorientation, or even coma, in someone with severe liver disease?

• The hepatitis B virus vaccine can be hailed as the first anticancer vaccine?

"Sanjiv Chopra is one of the most talented hepatologists in the field. He has an encyclopedic knowledge of medicine and possesses the clinical expertise to utilize it for the maximum benefit of his patients. He is also a charismatic teacher. This book is a testament to these skills. It completely demystifies liver disease for the nonphysician, and should be welcomed by everyone interested in the liver and its pathology."

—Robert C. Moellering Jr., M.D., physician in chief and chairman, Department of Medicine, Beth Israel Deaconess Medical Center, Harvard Medical School

DR. SANJIV CHOPRA'S
LIVER BOOK

A COMPREHENSIVE GUIDE TO DIAGNOSIS, TREATMENT, AND RECOVERY

Sanjiv Chopra, M.D.
with Sharon Cloud Hogan

A FIRESIDE BOOK
PUBLISHED BY SIMON & SCHUSTER
NEW YORK   LONDON   TORONTO   SYDNEY   SINGAPORE

The ideas, procedures, and suggestions in this book are not intended as a substitute for the medical advice of your trained health professional. All matters regarding your health require medical supervision. Consult your physician before adopting the suggestions in this book, as well as about any condition that may require diagnosis or medical attention. The author and publisher disclaim any liability arising directly or indirectly from the use of this book.

 Fireside
Rockefeller Center
1230 Avenue of the Americas
New York, NY 10020

Copyright © 2001 by Sanjiv Chopra

All rights reserved, including the right of reproduction in whole or in part in any form.

First Fireside Edition 2002

FIRESIDE and colophon are registered trademarks of
Simon & Schuster, Inc.

For information regarding special discounts for bulk purchases, please contact Simon & Schuster Special Sales at 1-800-456-6798 or business@simonandschuster.com

Designed by Stratford Publishing Services

Manufactured in the United States of America

10 9 8 7 6 5 4 3 2 1

ISBN 0-7434-2217-1
       0-7434-0584-4 (Pbk)

I dedicate this book to my patients and their families. Over the last quarter century, it has been my privilege to serve them. I have learned much from them about facing life with courage, fortitude, and humor. I shall cherish with gratitude the many lessons they have taught me.

Acknowledgments

I'm grateful to several of my colleagues at Boston's Beth Israel Deaconess Medical Center for their many valuable suggestions and contributions. In particular, Drs. Adam Silk and Booker Bush provided pertinent additions to the discussion of treatment for alcoholism. John Hogan shared his incredible ordeal with this common disease, as well as his inspirational story of how he finally conquered it.

Dr. Keith Stuart provided insights from a cancer specialist's perspective of liver tumors.

Drs. Maureen Martin, Elizabeth Pomfret, and Fredric Gordon contributed valuable and personal insights into what patients can expect when faced with a liver transplant.

I also would like to thank two liver transplant patients—Scott Jackle and Karen Scolaro—as well as a liver donor, Philip Scolaro. I admire the courage and honesty with which they were willing to talk about their experiences.

Not long ago, at a meeting in New Jersey, I spoke with Lucianna DiMeglio, a nurse who has had a lot of experience in the oncology arena and who now works with hepatitis C patients. She shared with me some tips on managing the side effects of interferon/ribavirin therapy.

I am also grateful to my agent, Lynn Franklin, for her guidance and support; to my editor at Pocket Books, Tracy Sherrod, for her enthusiasm and attention to detail; and to my publisher at Pocket Books, Judith Curr, for her vision.

Finally, I wish to express my deep appreciation and gratitude to Sharon Hogan, who worked tirelessly and diligently and researched some of the material for this book. She interviewed the people mentioned above and asked many probing questions of them and me. She helped me immensely in the writing of this book.

Contents

INTRODUCTION   xi

1. WHAT IS THE LIVER? WHAT DOES IT DO?   1

2. DIAGNOSING LIVER DISEASE   9

3. VIRAL HEPATITIS: FROM A TO G   21

4. HEPATITIS C: ARE YOU AT RISK?   55

5. HEPATITIS C: SYMPTOMS AND DIAGNOSIS   66

6. HEPATITIS C: TREATMENT   81

7. AUTOIMMUNE HEPATITIS   105

8. ALCOHOLIC LIVER DISEASE   117

9. CIRRHOSIS   147

10. PRIMARY BILIARY CIRRHOSIS   175

11. IRON OVERLOAD DISORDERS   194

12. LIVER TUMORS   211

13. LIVER TRANSPLANTS   235

CONCLUSION   269

NOTES TO SELECTED ARTICLES DESCRIBED IN THE TEXT   271

RESOURCES   273

INDEX   277

Introduction

Liver disease afflicts millions of people worldwide. It can range from a mild, reversible illness to advanced disease—often cirrhosis (severe scarring and distortion of the liver architecture)—with the potential for myriad and even life-threatening complications.

Many liver diseases occur in epidemic proportions. For example, 300 million individuals worldwide have chronic hepatitis B virus (HBV) infection; this is a mind-boggling 5% of the world population! Recent estimates suggest that 150 to 200 million people have chronic infection with the hepatitis C virus (HCV). The HCV epidemic has been called the "silent" or "shadow" epidemic because, although patients often are not aware that they are infected, they can be at risk for developing significant liver diseases, including cirrhosis and liver cancer.

Idiopathic genetic hemochromatosis, an inherited disorder in which excessive amounts of iron are deposited in many different parts of the body, including the liver, afflicts 1 in 300 individuals in the Caucasian population, particularly those of Celtic ancestry.

Alcoholic liver disease is another common disorder that affects millions of individuals from all walks of life. A liver disorder that on biopsy mimics alcoholic liver disease is also being recognized more and more. This condition, which is called nonalcoholic steatohepatitis (NASH), relates to diabetes and obesity—two very prevalent conditions in all parts of the world. The spectrum of liver injury associated with this disorder ranges from mild fatty infiltration and some inflammation of the liver to cirrhosis.

Truly remarkable and stupendous advances have been made in our understanding of many of these liver disorders. For example, the abnormal genes responsible for hemochromatosis and for a rarer liver disorder called Wilson's disease have been identified recently. Very important strides have also been made in our understanding of the epidemiology, natural history, diagnosis, and treatment of the major viruses that can affect the liver. Notably, liver transplantation has come of age. Technical advances in liver surgery, refinements in immunosuppressant drug therapy, and the use of living donors are exciting new developments as we enter the next millennium.

As we have developed a number of therapeutic options to treat many liver disorders, scientists also have addressed prevention of infection. Indeed, very effective vaccines exist to prevent both hepatitis A virus (HAV) and HBV infections. Since chronic HBV infection is linked to the development of primary liver cancer, from which 500,000 to 1 million people succumb each year, the HBV vaccine truly can be hailed as the first "anticancer" vaccine.

Authoritative and encyclopedic texts and innovative CD-ROM programs addressing the diverse, complex, and rapidly evolving discipline of hepatology are available for the medical professional. However, for patients and their families, these texts are of limited utility and often are difficult to interpret or understand. Many patients have tried to fill this void by surfing the Internet or World Wide Web in search of answers. Although this information is indeed easy to access, it can be inaccurate, ambiguous, or even misleading.

In this book, I have set out to explain the pivotal role of the liver as an ingenious engine that orchestrates in a masterful way the many functions that are vital for the sustenance of life. I've attempted to clarify the laboratory tests, diagnostic procedures, and treatment options available for the most common liver disorders. However, as in many other medical disciplines, advances in hepatology are made literally each day. Therefore the advice given in this book, although current at the time of this writing, will likely need to be updated as we increase our knowledge about liver disorders. I encourage you to see your internist or your gastroenterologist or hepatologist regularly and to check with him or her about the latest developments.

Finally, although the stories included in this book are those of actual patients, for the most part the names have been changed to protect their privacy. When real names are used, the individual has kindly granted permission to do so.

In conclusion, I hope that the information provided here will answer many of the questions that may linger in your mind after you have seen your internist or liver specialist. I hope that you find this book useful and that in some measure it contributes to maintaining or improving your health.

1

What Is the Liver?
What Does It Do?

There, inside, you filter and apportion
You separate and divide,
You multiply and lubricate
You raise and gather
The threads, the grams of life.
—PABLO NERUDA, "Ode to the Liver"

The liver is a powerful organ that has long been linked to human bravery, courage, and strength. People who are called chicken-livered or lily-livered are thought to be fainthearted and cowardly. Those possessed of a robust liver, in contrast, are thought to have both physical might and spiritual integrity. Indeed, the liver is considered by some to be the seat of the soul. In ancient times, augurs used animal organs to portend the future, and a deep red, healthy liver was an omen that all would be well. Today, with all of our scientific and medical advances and know-how, we still look to the liver as a measure of our vitality, for it has a unique and essential role in sustaining life.

If you've recently been diagnosed with a liver disease, you may be thinking about this all-important organ for the very first time. In this chapter, I'd like to share with you some basic details regarding where your liver is situated in your body and its essential functions. Once you

1

have a clear idea of what this organ is all about, in the next chapter I'll tell you what you can expect if you visit your primary care physician or liver specialist and you are told that something in your liver may have gone awry. Then, in the chapters that follow, you'll find a guide to the symptoms, diagnosis, and treatment of major liver diseases.

WHERE IS YOUR LIVER?

If you take your right forefinger and trace the bottom of your right rib cage, you're very close indeed to the bottom of your liver, which lies for the most part just beneath your lower ribs. The top of your liver is roughly at the level of your nipples. Situated in the right upper part of your abdomen, your liver is sheltered by your rib cage on the right side. It rests below your lungs and above your kidneys.

Beneath the liver is your gallbladder. This tiny pear-shaped, saclike organ receives bile, a yellowish green fluid that the liver produces to help digest and absorb fats. The gallbladder concentrates bile before passing it into the small intestine via a tube called the common bile duct.

Blood also travels through the liver in fairly copious amounts. About two-thirds of the liver's blood supply enters this organ through the portal vein; the remaining third arrives, well oxygenated, via the hepatic artery. *Hepatic* means liver, and the hepatic artery is the only artery that enters the liver from the aorta, which carries blood from the heart. As blood exits the liver, the hepatic veins carry it away to the right side of the heart.

WHAT IS THE LIVER LIKE?

Your liver is the largest organ in your body. It weighs about three pounds and in some people is about as large as a standard-size football. In adults it represents roughly one-fiftieth of total body weight; in infants it's relatively larger, comprising one-eighteenth of body weight.

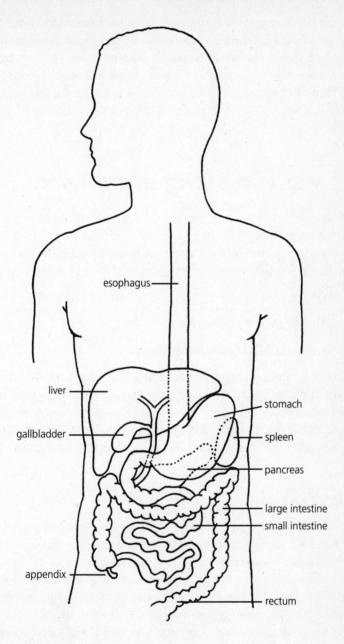

esophagus

liver

gallbladder

stomach

spleen

pancreas

large intestine

small intestine

appendix

rectum

Your liver is composed of two major lobes: a left lobe and a right lobe that is five to six times bigger than the left. These lobes are separated by a smooth membrane called the falciform ligament. On the outside, a healthy liver is smooth and reddish brown because of its rich blood supply. (In medical jargon, we would say that it's a very "vascular" organ.) On the inside, the liver consists of a busy and intricate network of ducts, veins, and liver cells. The liver cells are called hepatocytes.

WHY IS THE LIVER SO IMPORTANT?

A healthy liver, which is so critical to our well-being, is akin to a master conductor who is orchestrating a number of essential functions. It acts as a central manufacturing factory, toxic-waste-processing plant, and warehouse. It's also a site where many ingenious transformations occur.

THE LIVER AS A FACTORY

Albumin and blood-clotting proteins

The liver produces a major protein in the blood called albumin, which is key to regulating the fluid balance within our bodies. It is also the place where the major coagulation, or blood-clotting, factors are produced. In the next chapter, I'll tell you how doctors measure these proteins in your blood to determine how well your liver is functioning.

Bile

Throughout history, the connections that man has made between the liver and the human spirit have extended to one of this organ's important products: a substance called bile. People once spoke of "having bile" when they were referring to either a fiery temper or melancholia. Today the term is still used to mean an inclination to anger. Another term for bile, *gall,* has long been associated with wrath and rancor.

In truth, bile doesn't have anything to do with a sour mood. Rather, it's a fluid—consisting of water, bile salts, a pigment called bilirubin, and other substances—that is necessary for the breakdown of fats by the intestines. The liver produces bile continuously, and its flow to the intestines is very important. Blockage of the flow of bile can lead to a condition called cholestasis. This problem is associated with several disorders, including one called primary biliary cirrhosis, which I'll tell you about later in this book.

Urea

Ammonia is a chemical that is produced as a by-product of digestion. One of the liver's many tasks is to break this substance down. In doing so, it forms a waste product called urea. If the liver isn't functioning well, ammonia can build up in the body and can cause mental confusion.

THE LIVER AS AN INGENIOUS ENGINE THAT PERFORMS MAGIC

The liver magically transforms quite a number of substances such as cholesterol and fats into other substances. These "metabolic" processes result in the production of essential substances that the body needs as well as waste products that it can readily dispose of. Let's look more closely at the materials that the liver refashions.

Bilirubin

Red blood cells, which carry oxygen through your body, only live for 90 to 120 days. When they die, they release a pigment called bilirubin, which is taken up by the liver and metabolized into a water-soluble substance that is excreted in bile. The bile flows in the bile ducts and is transported into the intestines. Bilirubin breakdown is a normal activity of a healthy liver. If your liver is damaged and it fails to keep up with such tasks, this bile pigment can accumulate in your blood, causing your skin and the whites of your eyes to look yellow, or jaundiced.

Cholesterol

Your liver also synthesizes steroids, including cholesterol (a fatty sub-stance that can clog the arteries and is the main constituent of the major kinds of gallstones encountered in the West). Your liver is the sole organ that removes cholesterol from the body. Cholesterol within the liver is converted into bile acids (which are essential for fat digestion), bile salts, and phospholipids, which are fats that are essential for cell maintenance and important sources of fuel for the body.

Carbohydrate metabolism

The liver plays a pivotal role in maintaining blood sugar concentra-tions within a relatively narrow range. It transforms sugars such as galactose and fructose to another kind of sugar called glucose. Glucose, in turn, is converted to a substance called glycogen, which you might think of as a box that is used to store carbohydrate energy in the ware-house of the liver.

THE LIVER AS WAREHOUSE

In addition to its creative and transforming capacities, the liver serves as a storage place for extra amounts of energy and iron.

Energy

Glycogen, the storage unit of carbohydrate energy that I mentioned ear-lier, is housed in the liver. You may have heard of marathon runners who practice "carbo loading," or consumption of large amounts of car-bohydrates, such as bread and pasta, before a race. When they need a boost of energy, the glycogen is converted back to glucose and is sent to the muscles and other organs.

Iron

Lastly, most of the body's stores of iron are found in the liver. In a disorder known as iron overload, excessive amounts of this trace mineral are absorbed by the gastrointestinal tract and then deposited in the liver, where a buildup of too much iron can cause liver damage (see chapter 11).

THE LIVER AS A PURIFICATION PLANT

The last significant role of the liver that I'd like to tell you about is that of purification, or detoxification.

Bacteria

Blood flowing from your intestines into the liver is contaminated by bacteria. Inside the liver, cells called Kupffer cells filter and remove bacteria from your blood.

Ammonia

As I said earlier, ammonia, a toxic chemical produced in the intestines when we digest foods, finds its way to the liver, where it is converted to a substance called urea that can be excreted by the kidneys. If a diseased liver fails to purge this poison from the body, ammonia can build up in the blood and affect the central nervous system to the extent that it can cause sleepiness, confusion, and even coma.

Alcohol

As you'll read in chapter 8, alcohol, like many other toxins, is broken down and converted to other substances by your liver. In its attempts to clear this chemical from the body, the liver creates a substance called acetaldehyde. This by-product of alcohol metabolism can be quite damaging to liver cells.

Drugs

In addition to dangerous chemicals like ammonia and alcohol, the liver is responsible for "detoxifying" all kinds of drugs, including many antibiotics, sedatives, tranquilizers, and drugs used to lower cholesterol or thin the blood. If your liver is not functioning well, major drug reactions can occur.

Now that you know where the liver is located and how it functions when it's working properly, let's move on to chapter 2, where you'll find a brief run-through of what you can expect when you go to your doctor's office because of a liver problem.

2

. . . .

Diagnosing Liver Disease

You may be reading this book because you or someone you love has a liver disorder. This condition could be mild and reversible, or it could be more serious. Regardless of the severity of your liver disease, if you are ill and you go to see your primary care physician, she will begin to search for clues to the nature of your illness following a tried-and-true sequence of diagnostic steps. Likewise, if you go to see your doctor for an annual physical examination, she may become alerted to the possibility that you could have a liver problem because you have certain symptoms (such as nausea, flu-like symptoms, and mild abdominal discomfort) or clinical signs (such as flushed, red palms or red spiderlike veins at the surface of your skin). Last, in the absence of such clues, your physician may learn that you have liver disease by means of routine blood tests.

Regardless of how your liver problem is discovered, your doctor will try to gather more information and make a firm diagnosis with the help of certain diagnostic tests and procedures. At a certain point in this process, your primary care physician may refer you to a liver specialist (a hepatologist) or to a specialist in disorders of the gastrointestinal tract (a gastroenterologist) to confirm the diagnosis or to offer expert advice regarding the proper management of the liver (hepatic) problem.

In this chapter, you'll find an overview of the many procedures that you may encounter as well as advice about how you can plan and prepare for them.

HISTORY

When you go to visit your doctor, he undoubtedly will ask you a series of questions to get a sense of your medical history and the symptoms that have brought you to the examining room. Some seemingly "non-specific" symptoms (that is, symptoms that could relate to many different types of disorders) such as weakness, fatigue, and weight loss may actually be related to liver disease, so it's always important to bring them to your doctor's attention, even if you do not think they are important. Conversely, more specific symptoms commonly associated with liver disease, such as jaundice, can occasionally have nothing to do with a liver problem. (For instance, jaundice may be caused by malaria or a type of anemia called hemolytic anemia.)

Both nonspecific and specific symptoms are simply clues to your physician that you *might* have a liver disorder. He will need to do further tests to find out what's going on.

PHYSICAL EXAMINATION

When your doctor examines you, he may find certain medical signs, or objective characteristics, of a particular liver disorder. Throughout this book, when I use the term *sign,* I'll be referring to this type of feature. A *symptom,* in contrast, refers to a manifestation of an illness (such as fatigue, pain, or itching) that you, the patient, may be experiencing. Regardless of the severity of your illness, you may have some of these features of liver disease or you may have none at all. It's a good idea to be aware of them, however, so that you can inform your doctor if you notice any of these characteristics.

When I'm examining a patient who may have liver disease, these are the signs that I often look for:

- Skin problems linked with chronic liver disease, such as red palms and red, spiderlike veins on the surface of the skin (these are called spider telangiectasias, or spider nevi).
- Gynecomastia, or enlarged breasts in men. In certain liver conditions, gynecomastia may be accompanied by small or shrunken testes.

- Enlargement of the liver and spleen.
- A distended belly full of fluid (this is called ascites).
- Jaundice, or yellowing of the skin and the whites of the eyes.
- Features of hepatic encephalopathy. In cases of advanced liver disease, toxins such as ammonia can build up in the blood and lead to mental confusion. Patients with this condition can have "constructional apraxia," an inability to carry out certain motor activities such as writing one's name or drawing a picture of a star. Another sign of this condition is called a "flapping tremor." Doctors test for this by asking the patient to put his or her arms straight out, with the hands also held straight out and the fingers spread apart. With hepatic encephalopathy, both hands may "flap," usually not at the same time.

Patients with hepatic encephalopathy also may have fetor hepaticus, or "liver breath," a characteristic fruity, pungent, musty breath odor.

LABORATORY BLOOD TESTS

If your doctor is highly suspicious that you have liver disease because of specific clues from your history and physical exam, he or she may order blood tests to confirm a diagnosis. Also, if you have nonspecific symptoms (again, this means that they may be associated with many different conditions) such as weight loss and fatigue, your doctor may run blood tests including those to check for kidney and liver function, and in doing so may find that the results of your liver function tests (LFTs) are abnormal. Finally, some doctors check LFTs as part of a regular screening whenever their patients come in for a first visit or for a regular physical exam. This comprehensive health screening may be done and abnormal results may be detected even though your doctor began the workup with no suspicion that you had a liver disease.

These are the blood tests that are commonly performed:

- **Complete blood count (CBC).** This routine test will allow your doctor to see if you have an abnormal red blood cell count or white blood cell count. Patients with liver diseases usually have a normal or low red blood cell count (the latter condition is called anemia). The white blood cell count can be normal, low, or high. The CBC is not used alone to diagnose any one particular liver disorder; rather, taken together with other diagnostic tests, it helps to build a detailed clinical picture of a person's liver disease.

- **Liver function tests (LFTs).** The LFTs include tests for liver enzymes ALT and AST, alkaline phosphatase, bilirubin, albumin, prothrombin time, and lactate dehydrogenase.

   Liver enzymes. Two important liver enzymes are called alanine transaminase (ALT; also called serum glutamic pyruvic transaminase, or SGPT) and aspartate transaminase (AST; also called serum glutamic oxaloacetic transaminase, or SGOT). Both AST and ALT levels may be elevated with several liver disorders, because these enzymes are released from liver cells that die because of ongoing liver injury. The ALT and AST levels are extremely high (for instance, twenty times the upper limit of normal) with conditions such as acute viral hepatitis that can cause an acutely inflamed liver, or acute hepatocellular injury. Drug toxicity (due to many different medications including common ones such as acetaminophen, or Tylenol) can also lead to this type of injury.

   Although high liver enzyme levels can suggest liver disease, they may be elevated in certain muscle disorders also. Furthermore, levels of these two enzymes do not always relate directly to the degree of liver damage that your physician may discover if you undergo a liver biopsy.

   Alkaline phosphatase. High levels of a group of enzymes called alkaline phosphatase may provide a clue to the presence of certain liver diseases. Alkaline phosphatase levels are often high with both acute and chronic (or long-term) cholestatic liver disorders; that is, disorders caused by a blockage of bile flow within the liver or in the bile ducts leaving the liver and entering the small intestines. These disorders include primary biliary cirrhosis (PBC), primary sclerosing cholangitis (PSC), and a condition called intrahepatic cholestasis of pregnancy. Liver damage from certain drugs also may cause an elevation of the level of this liver enzyme.

   Although elevated alkaline phosphatase levels may signal the presence of a liver problem, it's important to keep in mind that high levels can be a normal phenomenon in healthy young people, because this enzyme is also present in bones and thus an elevated level is related to bone growth. The alkaline phosphatase normally is increased in healthy pregnant women, too.

Finally, your alkaline phosphatase level may be normal in spite of liver disease, so this test result is not considered in isolation.

Bilirubin. As I mentioned in chapter 1, bilirubin is a bile pigment that can build up in the blood because of certain liver disorders. A blood test to measure this bile pigment may or may not be an important prognostic indicator, though, because you may have a high bilirubin level with either mild or very severe disease.

Albumin. Likewise, levels of albumin, a protein that is synthesized in the liver, may be normal even though a person has acute liver disease. Levels of this protein may be low in a number of conditions, including cirrhosis of the liver; however, other things can cause a low albumin level too, including malnutrition and a variety of kidney and intestinal disorders.

Prothrombin time. Most blood-clotting factors are synthesized by the liver. A test called prothrombin time (PT) may be used to determine whether or not your liver is producing these blood-clotting factors adequately.

Acute liver injury can cause a prolonged PT. However, this abnormal result also is seen in patients who have a vitamin K deficiency, so if your PT is elevated, your doctor may give you an injection of vitamin K to correct this possible deficiency. If the PT remains elevated after this injection, you most likely have some form of liver disease.

Lactate dehydrogenase. Elevated levels of an enzyme called lactate dehydrogenase (LDH) also may be a clue to the presence of liver disease, especially if your alkaline phosphatase level is elevated too.

OTHER BLOOD TESTS

Once your doctor suspects or confirms that you have a liver disease, he may do further testing to determine the cause. I'll describe these special tests more fully throughout this book when I discuss the disorders that they relate to. For now, here's a brief overview:

- **Alpha-fetoprotein (AFP).** This blood test is used to screen for a type of liver tumor called primary hepatocellular carcinoma (also called hepatoma). Elevated AFP levels are also normal in benign conditions and during pregnancy, though, so having a high AFP level does not necessarily mean that you have liver cancer.
- **Serum ceruloplasmin.** If your doctor thinks that you may have a rare disorder called Wilson's disease, in which excessive amounts of copper accumulate in the body, he may likely test your serum ceruloplasmin level.
- **Antimitochondrial antibody (AMA)** is used to diagnose a disorder called primary biliary cirrhosis. I generally use this test if my patient has symptoms of this disorder (such as itching and fatigue), and the alkaline phosphatase level is high.
- **Antinuclear antibody (ANA)** is used to help diagnose a condition called autoimmune hepatitis.
- **Hepatitis viral serological markers** are blood tests to look for the hepatitis viruses. These tests include:

    HAV antibody. This test diagnoses hepatitis A virus (HAV) infection.

    HBV surface antigen and *HBV core antibody.* These tests diagnose hepatitis B virus (HBV) infection.

    HCV-RNA-PCR. This special quantitative test measures the amount of the hepatitis C virus (HCV) circulating in a person's blood.

- **HCV genotype testing.** There are several genetic strains, or genotypes, of HCV, so if you have this virus, your liver specialist will likely give you a blood test to determine which genotype of the virus you are infected with.
- **Iron studies** such as serum ferritin may be done to measure the amount of iron stored in your liver and your body. These levels may be low in people with iron deficiency (anemia) and high in people with an "iron overload" disorder (see chapter 11).

IMAGING TESTS

Different imaging tests such as computed axial tomographic (CAT) scans and magnetic resonance imaging (MRI) scans are useful for answering different questions. Each one also has potential advantages and disadvantages relative to the cost and the amount of radiation involved. Sometimes doctors use more than one test if questions remain after the first scan.

Here are the imaging tests that you may be asked to have:

• **Ultrasound.** An ultrasound test is a painless, inexpensive procedure that makes use of high-frequency sound waves. These sound waves are directed toward the area that needs to be viewed—in this case, your liver—and when they bounce off the internal structures of the body, they produce images that may reveal gallstones, a fluid buildup called ascites, or a liver tumor.

This is how it works: Before an ultrasound test to view your liver, a technician will apply a gel over your abdomen. Then he or she will move a device called a transducer over your abdomen, and images of your liver will be transmitted via the transducer to a video screen. Because this imaging test does not involve radiation, it is perfectly safe for patients who are pregnant and others for whom exposure to radiation may be a concern.

• **Computed axial tomography (CAT scan, also called a CT scan)** is sometimes used to look for telltale signs of liver scarring (cirrhosis); iron overload (one of the few causes of increased density of the liver tissue); and liver tumors. This test is not performed for patients who are pregnant, because small amounts of radiation are involved.

Like ultrasound, CAT is a painless technique that is used to obtain pictures of the liver. Unlike ultrasound, however, these images are reassembled to show "slices," or cross sections, of the liver.

A CAT scan generally is done while you are lying on a table or bed, and the radiologist moves the X-ray machine around you.

• **Magnetic resonance imaging (MRI)** is a good way to look for liver tumors and excessive amounts of iron in the liver. MRI is similar to CT, but it makes use of a magnet and a radio signal, rather than radiation, to create images of the body. If you are asked to undergo an MRI scan, you should be aware that this test will be done while you are lying inside a large, tubelike machine. If you are claustrophobic, you should let your doctor know.

• **Magnetic resonance angiography (MRA).** MRA is similar to MRI, but it is used specifically to view the blood flow within the liver. It provides excellent anatomical detail regarding the blood vessels of the liver and can be very useful as a "road map" for the liver surgeon.

• **Percutaneous transhepatic cholangiography (PTC).** PTC is a good test to determine what is causing a patient's jaundice. During PTC, a skilled radiologist inserts a needle into the liver and injects dye into the bile ducts. X-ray pictures then can be taken as the dye flows through the liver.

• **Endoscopic retrograde cholangiopancreatography (ERCP).** This test generally is done by a skilled gastroenterologist, who inserts a tube called an endoscope through the patient's mouth and down the esophagus. A catheter then is inserted where the bile duct opens into the intestine (this is called the ampulla). Just as with PTC, a dye is injected and X-ray pictures are taken.

• **Magnetic resonance cholangiopancreatography (MRCP).** MRCP is a new, noninvasive technique for evaluating the pancreatic duct and the bile ducts both inside and outside the liver. Unlike ERCP, no contrast material is administered before this test.

• **Hepatic scintiscanning.** This test, also called a technetium sulfur colloid scan, or a liver-spleen scan, is seldom done, but I find it useful in some circumstances, especially if I think my patient may have a condition called focal nodular hyperplasia (FNH) (see pages 223–25). This test uses very small amounts of a radioactive tracer called technetium to view the liver and spleen. This tracer is given intravenously before the test; when it is taken up by the liver, the radiation that it emits can be recorded by an imaging device.

• **Hepato-iminodiacetic acid (HIDA) scan.** A HIDA scan is similar to a technetium scan, except that it uses a different isotope, rather than technetium, as a radioactive tracer.

If one of my patients has abdominal pain with or without fever, and I'm concerned that he or she has acute cholecystitis (a condition in which a gallstone has blocked a duct called the cystic duct through

which the bile flows out of the gallbladder into the common bile duct),
I may request a HIDA scan.

LIVER BIOPSY

The most definitive way of diagnosing and confirming various types of
liver diseases is by performing a liver biopsy. In addition to its diagnostic value, a liver biopsy is useful for confirming the stage or degree of
disease and for excluding other diseases that may be contributing to the
abnormal results of your liver function tests. For example, in many
chronic liver conditions, a biopsy allows us to ascertain whether severe
liver scarring, or cirrhosis, has developed or not.

A biopsy also can help us to exclude other coexisting liver disorders.
For instance, I recently saw a patient with chronic HBV infection. She
was overweight, and her LFTs were abnormal. A biopsy showed that a
condition called nonalcoholic steatohepatitis (NASH), rather than HBV,
was causing her liver damage.

NEEDLE BIOPSY

An overwhelming majority (more than 95 percent) of patients who
undergo a liver biopsy have a relatively simple outpatient procedure
called a percutaneous needle biopsy. This procedure, which often is
done by a hepatologist or gastroenterologist, sounds unpleasant and
scary, but it's generally not painful (in some patients it produces discomfort). Another key thing to remember is that this procedure has an
extremely low complication rate and will not adversely affect the function of your liver.

I advise my patients who are preparing for a percutaneous liver
biopsy not to take any iron supplements, aspirin, ibuprofen, or other
"blood-thinning" products for ten days before the biopsy. It's generally
okay to take limited amounts of acetaminophen (Tylenol) for pain during this time, but do check with your doctor. You also shouldn't have
anything to drink or eat after midnight the night before your biopsy.

When you go to the hospital for this procedure, a nurse will greet you,
take a very brief history, and will record your baseline vital signs. The
doctor then will offer you mild sedation. Usually only half of my patients

choose sedation (5 to 10 mg of Valium by mouth). Although the idea of a liver biopsy may be unsettling to you (and you may say, "Please knock me out"), your doctor won't give you very strong sedation because you will need to be awake enough to hold your breath briefly while the biopsy is being performed.

During the procedure your physician first will percuss, or "tap out," your liver, and mark a suitable spot. An ultrasound probe will be used to confirm that the spot chosen for the liver biopsy is indeed appropriate. The surface of your skin will then be cleansed with an antiseptic solution, and a local anesthetic agent will be injected. This injection can feel like a bee sting, but the discomfort is transient. Your liver specialist then will obtain a liver sample by inserting a needle into your liver for a second or so while you are holding your breath.

After this tiny piece of liver tissue has been taken out, a small bandage will be used to cover up the area. You won't need stitches, and this procedure most often doesn't leave a noticeable scar. Some of my patients experience discomfort at the biopsy site and at the right shoulder. The latter is called "referred pain." If you are uncomfortable, you will receive two extra-strength tablets of Tylenol with or without codeine.

We monitor patients in the hospital for about four hours before they can go home. At our hospital, patients are required to have someone accompany them home after a biopsy is performed. I tell my patients that they can resume their normal activities within two or three days after this procedure.

As I mentioned earlier, complications from needle biopsies are rare. Significant bleeding occurs only in about 1 in 500, and 999 out of 1,000 patients will not require a transfusion because of procedure-related bleeding. Fatal complications are *extremely rare* and are said to be in the vicinity of 1 in 5,000 to 10,000 patients. I've been very fortunate in that none of my patients have had a fatal complication from a liver biopsy, although I have done several thousands of these procedures.

TRANSVENOUS BIOPSY

If you have severe abdominal swelling ("tense ascites") or a markedly increased risk for bleeding, your hepatologist may choose not to take the risks associated with a needle biopsy and may recommend that another route altogether be taken to obtain that important bit of liver tissue.

This procedure, known as transvenous or transjugular biopsy, is seldom done in community hospitals, and even in large academic centers it isn't commonly performed.

During this procedure, a radiologist will guide a small device through the internal jugular vein in your neck and then direct it to the hepatic vein within your liver. A tiny needle will then be inserted through the device and into the liver to capture a small biopsy specimen.

SURGICAL BIOPSY

Sometimes if my patient has a liver problem such as chronic HCV infection or abnormal LFT blood tests and he also needs to have an operation for another reason (such as to remove a diseased gallbladder or kidney), I ask the surgeon to take a liver biopsy while the patient is undergoing an open abdominal operation (laparoscopy or laparotomy).

READING THE RESULTS OF YOUR BIOPSY

No matter how your biopsy sample was obtained, your results probably will be available in a couple of days. Your physician can help you to interpret the pathologist's report, but here are some guidelines. In patients with chronic viral hepatitis, liver pathologists currently use a staging system (on a scale of 0 to 4) to indicate how inflamed the liver tissue is. More important, they grade the amount of scar tissue on a scale of 0 to 4. Patients who have grade 3 or 4 fibrosis, or scar tissue, have fairly advanced liver disease. Grade 4 fibrosis is synonymous with cirrhosis of the liver.

ENDOSCOPY

If your liver biopsy reveals advanced liver disease (cirrhosis), your gastroenterologist or hepatologist will likely recommend that you undergo a procedure called an upper endoscopy to look for engorged veins (varices) in your esophagus. Varices are a serious consequence of liver disease because ruptured varices can lead to severe and potentially fatal bleeding.

To prepare for an endoscopy, do not take any iron supplements, aspirin, ibuprofen, or other anti-inflammatory drugs for ten days before the procedure. You should also tell your doctor if you have a known heart murmur or artificial joints, if you take an anticoagulant drug such as warfarin (Coumadin), and if you normally take antibiotics before you undergo dental work.

For this procedure, you will be given a topical anesthetic and adequate intravenous sedation. A gastroenterologist or hepatologist will insert a flexible fiber-optic instrument through your mouth and into your esophagus and stomach. Like the liver biopsy, this is a very simple test with an extremely low complication rate. When I do this procedure, if I find that my patient has varices, I often prescribe a drug called propranolol (Inderal). This drug, which also is used to treat high blood pressure, or hypertension, decreases the risk of bleeding from varices. At our hospital we recommend that patients have someone accompany them home approximately one and one-half hours after the procedure.

SUMMARY

In general, the diagnosis of liver disease is not very difficult. Doctors diagnose liver disease by taking a person's history to learn about symptoms and by means of simple, usually quite routine blood tests. These tests can be done in any standard laboratory or hospital-affiliated lab. If you require sophisticated blood tests (for example, to measure the amount of hepatitis C virus circulating in your blood via a test called HCV-RNA-PCR), your doctor may send a blood sample to a specialized lab.

Once this initial evaluation has been completed and your doctor determines that you have a liver disease, he or she may refer you to a gastroenterologist or a hepatologist. That specialist will decide about which further tests are needed. He or she may recommend a liver biopsy, a simple outpatient procedure that has a low risk of complications.

Now that you are familiar with how doctors diagnose liver disorders, let's explore the major forms of liver disease, as well as the additional tests that may be used to assess them and the types of treatments available.

3

Viral Hepatitis: From A to G

I run a printing company, and last month I had to fly to Chicago on business. On the plane I read an article in a news magazine about hepatitis C. I was surprised to read that a person could be walking around with hepatitis C infection without knowing it, and that it's possible to get hepatitis C by snorting cocaine.

I'm thirty-seven years old and I think of myself as being in good health. I only tried coke a few times when I was in college in the early 1980s, and I've never used intravenous drugs, but this article left me wondering.

A few days after returning home, I went to my doctor and requested a blood test, and guess what—it was positive! I'm completely blown away. I don't even know what hepatitis really is—and I'm scared.

If your doctor tells you that you have hepatitis, she means that your liver has been damaged somehow, and it's not perfectly healthy. *Hepar* is Greek for "liver," and the word *hepatitis* literally means "inflammation of the liver," just as *tonsillitis* means "inflammation of the tonsils" and *arthritis* means "inflammation of the joints."

Viral hepatitis is usually caused by one of five different hepatitis viruses (A, B, C, D, or E). There are other, nonviral causes of hepatitis too. If you drink a lot of alcohol, for instance, you may be at risk for a serious and potentially fatal form of liver disease called alcoholic hepatitis. Rarely, even commonly used medicines can produce what is called drug-induced hepatitis. Conditions such as autoimmune hepatitis, a rare disease that involves intolerance to one's own liver cells, and nonalcoholic steatohepatitis (NASH), a liver injury that resembles that caused by alcohol, also can cause the liver to become inflamed.

I'll talk more about these other causes of hepatitis in chapters 7 and 8. In this chapter I'll describe only those forms of hepatitis that are caused by the major viruses affecting the liver.

ACUTE VS. CHRONIC HEPATITIS

Your physician may characterize your case of viral hepatitis as being either acute or chronic. *Acute* hepatitis simply means inflammation of the liver due to some form of insult that occurred in the very recent past. This liver injury, which may be caused by a drug, toxin, or virus, most often occurs only days or weeks before you and your doctor realize that you have hepatitis.

If you have acute hepatitis, you may or may not have a flulike illness and jaundice, a condition that can make your skin and the whites of your eyes look yellow. Although many people equate jaundice with hepatitis, jaundice can be due to other causes, and hepatitis can occur without jaundice. An acute episode of hepatitis lasts a few weeks, or at most a few months. If the episode was due to either the hepatitis A or B virus, chances are very good that you will recover without any long-term ill effects. Unfortunately, with acute hepatitis C virus infection, it's a different story.

Chronic hepatitis means that the infection will last at least six months. In reality, this infection is often lifelong.

The hepatitis A, B, C, D, and E viruses can all cause acute hepatitis, but only hepatitis B, C, and D can lead to chronic hepatitis. Among these viruses, hepatitis C has the greatest likelihood of becoming chronic. In fact, of all adults who get acute hepatitis C, 70 to 80 percent go on to develop chronic infection. In contrast, less than 5 percent of adults who get acute hepatitis B go on to develop chronic infection.

OTHER NAMES FOR VIRAL HEPATITIS INFECTIONS

If you have chronic viral hepatitis and you're reading everything you can find about your disease, you may come across some perplexing terms for your infection. In particular, we used to divide long-term cases of hepatitis into two categories: chronic persistent (also called persistent hepatitis) or chronic active (also called aggressive hepatitis). The implication was that chronic persistent hepatitis was a benign condition that wouldn't progress to scarring of the liver, or cirrhosis. In contrast, the terms *chronic active* and *aggressive* hepatitis suggested a more serious form of the disease that might evolve into cirrhosis and its complications.

For the most part, these confusing terms are being abandoned. Indeed, an international society has recommended that pathologists (specialists who interpret the results of various biopsy tests) not use these terms when evaluating liver biopsy results for the simple reason that the "benign" chronic persistent hepatitis can progress to the "more advanced" chronic active or aggressive hepatitis.

So, keep in mind that after you are diagnosed with a certain kind of viral hepatitis (such as hepatitis A or hepatitis B), *acute* and *chronic* are really the only labels that you'll need. If you have chronic hepatitis, a liver biopsy will reveal the extent of your liver damage. It may show mild or in some cases advanced disease—cirrhosis of the liver.

HEPATITIS A VIRUS

Let's talk now about the different kinds of hepatitis viruses. In the United States, the *hepatitis A virus (HAV)* is responsible for one-fourth of all cases of viral hepatitis. This virus generally causes a very mild and short-lived illness, even without treatment. Fatalities from HAV infection rarely occur.

Are You at Risk?

Throughout the world, HAV often is spread through impure food and water in overcrowded places where there are poor standards of personal hygiene. In this country, contaminated food has been implicated in more than thirty outbreaks of HAV infection since 1983. Such outbreaks sometimes occur when people eat food such as lettuce, strawberries, and shellfish that originated in unsanitary areas.

Although it's possible to become infected with HAV by eating an innocent-looking strawberry in Michigan or New Mexico, your risk of contracting this virus from contaminated food and water is much higher if you travel to countries where HAV is prevalent or if you live or work in an overcrowded environment or epidemic-prone community.

This virus also may be spread by fecal contamination and—rarely—by infected blood. The practice of oral-anal sex and the use of intravenous drugs may put you at risk.

Prevention

THE HAV VACCINE. We're very fortunate to have an effective vaccine that can prevent HAV infection in adults and children over the age of two. Two doses of this vaccine (one dose followed by a booster dose six months later) can confer protection from HAV infection for ten to twenty years.

Children who are younger than two years old who are at risk of contracting HAV may be given immune globulin to prevent infection.

SHOULD YOU BE VACCINATED? Whether or not you should be vaccinated against HAV depends in part on whether you have been exposed to this virus either in the remote or recent past. If so, you may have been infected and recovered—even without knowing it. If your body has ever initiated an immune response to the virus, your blood will still carry telltale antibodies that will provide you with lifelong protection from HAV—and you don't need to get vaccinated. A simple blood test can tell your doctor whether or not you're already immune.

In major metropolitan centers in this country, approximately half of all people fifty years of age or older have detectable antibodies to HAV. In many other parts of the world, such as Mexico, Costa Rica, Belgium, India, and Israel, about 90 percent of the population have been exposed to HAV and have developed antibodies to this virus by early adulthood.

Improved sanitation and hygiene practices in the United States have prevented many people from exposure to HAV at an early age, when they might have built up immunity to this disease. HAV infection in children is often mild, but in adults it can be quite severe. The paradox is that we encounter fewer patients with HAV in developed countries, but when we do so, they are often quite ill. Thus, I'm seeing more and more adult patients who have developed a pretty severe and debilitating bout of HAV infection.

If you're not immune to this virus, should you be vaccinated? We don't recommend universal immunization against HAV because the risk of contracting it from food and water is really very low in the United States. That said, the U.S. Centers for Disease Control (CDC) does advise some individuals to be vaccinated for the following reasons:

- **If you're a food handler.** You should be vaccinated if you work in a restaurant or food-processing facility, because if you acquire HAV infection you may spread this disease to others.
- **If you plan to travel to areas where HAV is common.** Quite often I see patients who are stricken with HAV infection while traveling in or shortly after returning from places where HAV is prevalent, or "endemic." If they are seasoned travelers, they may have been very careful before their first trip or two, and a few years ago (before a vaccine was available) they may have taken gamma globulin prophylaxis to protect themselves from contracting this virus. Sometimes, though, people are a little more casual or cavalier in preparing for subsequent journeys, and so they may have skipped such preventive measures and then, unfortunately, come down with HAV.

The CDC recommends that you receive the HAV vaccine if you're traveling to Africa, Asia (except Japan), the Mediterranean basin, Eastern Europe, the Middle East, Mexico, Central and South America, or the Caribbean.

- **Your children may need to be vaccinated if you live in certain states.** It may be wise to vaccinate your children if you live in states with at least 20 cases of HAV infection per 100,000 people (this is twice the national average). The states with this higher incidence of HAV are in the West: Arizona, Alaska, California, Idaho, Nevada, New Mexico, Oklahoma, Oregon, South Dakota, Utah, and Washington.
- **If you live or work in a crowded or epidemic-prone place.** Outbreaks of HAV have been known to occur in prisons, housing projects,

child care centers, and other facilities where there may be overcrowding. Some communities also have high rates of HAV infection and periodic epidemics, or sudden outbreaks of the virus. Native Alaskan, Hasidic Jewish, and some Hispanic communities, as well as American Indians living on reservations, have been known to experience outbreaks of HAV infection.

• **If you engage in oral-anal sexual activity.** Although most cases of HAV infection result from contaminated food and water, this pathogen also can be spread via infected stools. Thus, you may be at risk for developing HAV infection if you are a homosexual man or a person who has many sex partners and you have oral-anal sexual contact with a person who has HAV.

• **If you're exposed to HAV in the clinic or laboratory.** You should be vaccinated against HAV if you're a health care or research worker who may come into contact with the virus or if you work in a zoo or laboratory where there are nonhuman primates (like chimpanzees) who may carry the virus.

• **If you use intravenous drugs.** When a person is infected with HAV, the virus may be present in his bloodstream for a few days to a few weeks, and so he could give the virus to others if he shares intravenous needles during this time. Thus, if you're a street drug user, you should be vaccinated against HAV.

• **If you have other liver diseases.** Although other liver diseases do not cause you to be at a greater risk of getting HAV infection, if you have a chronic liver disease (for example, chronic HBV or HCV infection), you should be vaccinated against HAV. That's because if you get HAV infection on top of your already-existing liver disease, the consequences can be dire. If you've been diagnosed with such a disease, ask your doctor if you're susceptible to HAV. If so, you should receive the HAV vaccine.

Symptoms

If you haven't been exposed to HAV in childhood and you haven't been immunized against it, you could be unlucky and become infected.

In most people, HAV infection is a mild disorder that comes on quickly. You may develop a fever, a vague feeling of physical discomfort (malaise), and a loss of appetite. Your urine may darken and your feces may lighten a few days before the onset of jaundice. Often, if jaundice begins, these other symptoms subside. In addition to these common symptoms of HAV, some patients who smoke suddenly find cigarettes distasteful.

Approximately 10 percent of people who contract HAV infection are also at risk for developing an unusual variant of this illness called cholestatic hepatitis, which is characterized by deep jaundice and severe itching.

Diagnosis

PHYSICAL EXAMINATION. Most people who have HAV infection have such a minor illness that they don't even seek medical attention, so their infection is never diagnosed. However, if you experience any of the symptoms that I just described, you should go to your primary care physician to find out what's going on. She probably will find that you have an enlarged liver. If you are infected with HAV, there is also about a 1 in 3 chance that you have an enlarged spleen. There also may be abnormal enlargement of your lymph nodes.

LABORATORY TESTS. In addition to your physical examination, your doctor will draw a battery of blood tests. Some internists and family practitioners check these blood tests routinely whenever they see a patient for the first time during an office visit or when a patient has an annual physical examination.

Your physician will be able to tell if you have acute hepatitis if the level of liver enzymes—alanine transaminase (ALT) and aspartate transaminase (AST)—are strikingly elevated in your blood. If your liver is enlarged and the results of your liver enzyme tests are abnormal, your physician next will try to determine if hepatitis A is the culprit that's causing your liver to be inflamed. She can do so by checking another blood sample to see whether or not you have antibodies to the virus. If the results of this blood test, which is called the IgM anti-HAV antibody test, are positive, you definitely have HAV infection.

Usually no other tests are required if this antibody test is positive. Your doctor will not need to do radiologic studies such as computed axial tomographic (CAT) and magnetic resonance imaging (MRI) scans or a liver biopsy to establish this diagnosis. At this point, your physician may refer you to a specialist who handles problems of the gastrointestinal system (a gastroenterologist) or the liver (a hepatologist).

Treatment

If your antibody test is positive and your doctor tells you that you have HAV infection, what happens next? If you have a mild case of the disease, you may not need to do anything in terms of medical treatment. You should simply get plenty of rest and drink lots of fluids. Your jaundice probably will disappear on its own within a few weeks, and you most likely will recover completely within six months. However, in rare instances in which patients have intolerable symptoms such as itching due to cholestatic hepatitis, I sometimes prescribe a short course of steroid treatment with a drug called prednisone. This medicine is given for a few weeks to a month and can shorten the duration of the illness significantly.

In very rare circumstances, I encounter a patient with a severe case of HAV infection. He might have "fulminant hepatitis"; that is, acute liver failure that is preventing this organ from clearing toxins such as ammonia from the body. When these toxins reach the brain, mental confusion, drowsiness, stupor, and even coma can occur. Such patients should be referred to a center that can perform a liver transplant, which is the only treatment for this serious condition. Liver transplants are described in detail in chapter 13.

Are You Contagious?

If you've been diagnosed with HAV infection, you may wonder whether or not your family members and others close to you should be screened for the virus.

That depends. Your risk of spreading HAV to others is highest *before* you develop symptoms; once you develop jaundice, the risk of transmission wanes rapidly. Thus, if you've had intimate contact with anyone in the weeks before you developed symptoms, that person or persons should get a blood test to see if they are susceptible or immune to the virus. Studies have shown that for those individuals who are not immune, gamma globulin prophylaxis, when given within two weeks of a person's exposure to the virus, is effective in preventing HAV infection more than 90 percent of the time.

HEPATITIS B VIRUS

Like HAV, infection with the *hepatitis B virus (HBV)* is very preventable with a vaccine. The challenge is to make sure that all young people on this planet get inoculated, because there are an estimated 300 million "chronic carriers" of the virus—that's an extraordinary 5 percent of the world population! The prevalence of HBV is especially high in parts of Southeast Asia and sub-Saharan Africa.

HBV is also similar to HAV in that it usually doesn't cause severe illness. About 90 to 95 percent of adult patients with acute HBV infection recover completely. Less than 1 percent of adults with HBV have severe, fulminant hepatitis, and the risk of dying from a severe bout of acute HBV infection is also about 1 percent.

Two to 5 percent of adults who contract acute HBV infection will go on to have long-term, or chronic, HBV infection. They often are referred to as "chronic carriers." This means that the hepatitis B surface antigen (a marker of the virus) will persist in their blood for longer than six months. In reality, it often persists indefinitely.

If you are a chronic carrier, you may or may not have or develop symptoms of liver disease. Some patients can live a perfectly healthy life. Other patients develop mild liver injury; still others have liver damage that may range from liver scarring (cirrhosis) to liver cancer. Your chance of developing cirrhosis and liver cancer is especially great if you were infected with HBV during infancy or early childhood and you became a chronic carrier of the virus.

Are You at Risk?

The hepatitis B virus is present in high concentrations in the blood as well as in body fluids and secretions, including semen, saliva, tears, colostrum, and breast milk, so you may become infected if you are a health care worker and you accidentally stick yourself with a contaminated syringe, if you have sex with an infected person, or if you get a tattoo or acupuncture from a practitioner who is using unclean needles. This virus also can be transmitted from infected mothers to their infants during childbirth. Although children rarely develop severe liver disease because of HBV infection, a newborn who becomes infected with HBV has a 90 percent chance of becoming chronically infected with the virus. It's estimated that decades later, up to half of these children will go on to die of complications of cirrhosis or liver cancer.

Thus, if you're pregnant, you should be screened for HBV. (In the United States, this screening test is done for all pregnant women as part of routine prenatal care.) If you are found to be positive for the virus, your newborn should receive both the HBV vaccine and a special kind of gamma globulin called hepatitis B immune globulin (HBIG). The HBV vaccine and HBIG can be given simultaneously and should be administered within twelve hours of the child's birth.

Prevention

If you have one of the risk factors for HBV, your physician can give you the very effective HBV vaccine. This vaccine, which was approved by the U.S. Food and Drug Administration (FDA) in 1981, holds great promise for eradicating or significantly curtailing HBV infection on a worldwide basis. It also has been hailed as the first "anticancer" vaccine, because chronic HBV infection can lead to a type of liver cancer called hepatoma, or primary hepatocellular carcinoma.

Fortunately, "universal" HBV vaccination is now the rule in several countries. In many parts of the world, pharmaceutical companies have joined forces with the government to make the vaccine available for approximately $5 to $10. In contrast, the three-dose form of HBV vaccine that is given in the United States currently costs between $100 and $150. I'm hopeful that in the next few years it will cost considerably less, and that in the near future all newborns or young children worldwide will be vaccinated.

Symptoms

If you have HBV infection and your infection is *acute,* chances are you will be unwell, and you will go to see your doctor. You may feel fatigued or nauseous, and you may have no appetite. Your skin and the whites of your eyes may look yellow because of mild jaundice. Occasionally patients also develop a rash or joint pain. In contrast, if you have *chronic* HBV infection, you may or may not be experiencing any symptoms. If you are, they may range in severity from mild fatigue to abdominal pain and weight loss.

If your disease has progressed to an advanced stage, you may have developed liver scarring (cirrhosis) and its complications. You may find that you are retaining fluid in your abdomen (this is called ascites—pronounced "a-SITE-ease"), or you may bleed from engorged veins called varices in your esophagus. Both of these conditions, which are discussed in greater detail in chapter 9, require immediate medical attention.

Diagnosis

The diagnosis of HBV infection is similar to that of HAV infection. Your physician may find that your liver and spleen are enlarged, and blood tests will show that your liver enzyme levels (ALT and AST) are elevated.

THE DIAGNOSIS OF ACUTE HBV INFECTION. Once your doctor becomes aware that you have some type of liver inflammation (because he or she finds that your liver is enlarged and your ALT and AST levels are abnormal), the diagnosis of HBV infection can be confirmed with specific blood tests. If your disease is acute, a test called IgM anti-HBc (also called the IgM core antibody) will be positive. Another blood test, HBs Ag, usually is positive also. This test looks for something called the hepatitis B surface antigen, which is present in the blood early on in acute HBV infection, but then can disappear. If you are tested after the surface antigen has disappeared from your bloodstream, this test result may be negative even though you have an acute HBV infection and you are contagious. For this reason, doctors don't rely on the results of the surface antigen test alone.

Also, even if your blood is positive for the hepatitis B surface antigen, you may not have an acute HBV infection at all, but rather a *chronic* HBV infection with another acute viral infection (such as acute hepatitis A or C) or a case of drug-induced hepatitis "superimposed" on your chronic HBV infection. Many different things could be going on in a chronically infected person that may look like acute hepatitis B. Therefore, if the surface antigen test result is positive, the core antibody blood test should be done as well to confirm the diagnosis. Radiologic studies such as CT and MRI and a liver biopsy will not be necessary to confirm the diagnosis of acute HBV infection.

If your acute HBV infection is particularly severe, your doctor may test your blood to see if you also are infected with the hepatitis D (or "delta") virus, which can act as a "piggyback" virus to HBV. Although there is no proven treatment for HDV infection, determining whether or not you have HDV may explain the severity of your disease.

THE DIAGNOSIS OF CHRONIC HBV INFECTION. If your disease is chronic, both the IgG core antibody and the hepatitis B surface antigen blood tests will be positive. Your physician also may check your blood for evidence of HDV if you have chronic HBV infection, especially if your condition is getting worse. Again, coinfection with the delta virus would account for the severity of your illness. Knowledge of this infection also may influence your doctor's expectation of your treatment, because patients with both chronic HBV and HDV infection tend to have a poorer response to a drug called interferon (for more information about this drug, see pages 35–42) than those who are infected only with chronic HBV.

Once she has established the diagnosis of chronic HBV (and possibly HDV) infection by means of these blood tests, your doctor may refer you to a gastroenterologist or hepatologist for further evaluation and treatment. When you visit such a specialist, he probably will recommend that you undergo a liver biopsy to "stage" your disease, or determine how advanced it is. If you have chronic HBV, your risk of developing liver scarring, or cirrhosis, is approximately 25 percent. A liver biopsy will clarify whether the infection has damaged your liver to that extent. During this simple procedure, usually performed on an outpatient basis, your gastroenterologist or hepatologist will use a needle to procure a small piece of liver tissue, which then can be viewed under a microscope. Chapter 2 describes this procedure, and what you can do to prepare for it, in more detail.

Are You Contagious?

In patients with HBV infection, one can find the virus in virtually all of the body fluids, including semen, saliva, breast milk, and tears, and it is often present in huge amounts. Therefore this disease is highly contagious, and if you have a confirmed case of either acute or chronic HBV infection, members of your household should be screened for viral markers by having a blood test performed. Those who are found to be at risk should be vaccinated.

Treatment for Acute HBV Infection

Just as with acute HAV infection, there is no medical treatment for most cases of acute HBV. Your doctor probably will advise you to rest and drink plenty of fluids (except for alcoholic drinks, which can cause serious damage to your inflamed liver). If you follow these recommendations, you most likely will recover on your own within a short period of time. In rare instances (approximately 1 percent of cases), however, patients with acute HBV develop severe, fulminant hepatitis for which a liver transplant is the only therapeutic option. This lifesaving operation is described in chapter 13. Finally, as I mentioned earlier, if you have acute HBV infection there is a low (2 to 5 percent) risk of your disease becoming chronic. Ask your doctor about whether or not this appears to be a concern in your case. If it is, effective treatments are available.

Treatment for Chronic HBV Infection

If you've been diagnosed with chronic HBV infection, your gastroenterologist or hepatologist will oversee your treatment. When you go to see such a specialist, you may want to take along the list provided on page 44 as a reminder of important questions to ask.

SPECIAL PRECAUTIONS

ALCOHOL. Your liver specialist almost certainly will tell you that you must stop drinking alcohol, because alcohol may make the hepatitis B virus multiply more quickly, "accelerate" your liver disease, and put you at risk for serious complications such as cirrhosis. Aside from the damage that this chemical can do in relationship to your HBV infection, alcohol can suppress your immune system and, if taken in large amounts, cause injury in its own right (for example, it may lead to a condition called alcoholic liver disease; see chapter 8).

SCREENING FOR LIVER CANCER. Even though your risk of developing primary liver cancer (hepatoma) from HBV infection is very small, your doctor probably will screen you for it periodically. This screening usually entails ultrasound examinations of the liver and a blood test called alpha-fetoprotein (AFP). These regular tests are important, because early detection will increase the likelihood that a tumor can be removed successfully. To learn more about primary liver cancer, turn to chapter 12.

DRUG THERAPY

In the past, drugs used in an attempt to treat chronic HBV infection included corticosteroids, *Phyllanthus amarus* (a plant derivative used in ancient Indian medicine for centuries), and an "immunopotentiator" called levamisole, which was prescribed to stimulate the body's immune response. If you are diagnosed with HBV today, you probably will be given either of two effective medicines: interferon or lamivudine. The decision about which treatment option is best for you should be made by an experienced hepatologist.

INTERFERON. In 1957, two researchers at London's National Institute for Medical Research discovered that chicken cells were capable of producing a protein that could inhibit viral infection in other cells. They called this substance interferon because it "interferes" with the replication of viruses.

The human body also produces small amounts of interferon to fight viral, bacterial, and parasitic infections. Because this substance can interfere with cell division, it may slow the proliferation of cancer cells, too. Our bodies can't manufacture enough interferon to combat infections like hepatitis or diseases like multiple sclerosis or cancer, so doctors sometimes prescribe this drug to give the immune system more firepower. Interferon is sold under the trade names Intron A, Roferon A, and Infergen. At the time of this writing, there is no compelling evidence that any one of these products is superior to the others. The typical dosages of interferon for treatment of chronic HBV infection are 5 million units per day, or 10 million units three times per week. The average course of interferon treatment for HBV lasts 4 months.

If you have chronic HBV infection, you probably have many questions about this treatment option.

Can I take interferon? Before you start taking interferon, your doctor will draw your blood to check the counts of three important blood components:

- Your white blood cells (WBC), which are crucial for fighting infections
- Your hematocrit, or the volume of red blood cells in whole blood
- Your platelets, unique structures in your blood that help with blood clotting

Interferon has a predictable depressive effect on the bone marrow, which is the factory that produces these blood components, so all of these counts can fall in patients who take this drug. If you start off with counts that are already very low, then further bone marrow suppression can put you at risk for infections, bleeding, and anemia.

If your WBC count is lower than 3,000, for example, then you should be cautious about the use of interferon, because an even lower count can increase the chance that you may acquire an infection. Likewise, if you have a low red blood cell count and you take interferon, you could develop fatigue and shortness of breath—the side effects of anemia. A blood hemoglobin level under 10 grams per deciliter is considered to be low (the normal range is 13–15 g/dl). If your platelet count is less than 50,000, you probably won't be a candidate for interferon therapy, because if your platelet count drops any further, you may have an increased bleeding tendency.

If your counts are in an acceptable range, though, you can begin taking interferon, and your specialist will pay particular attention to these three counts while you are taking this drug.

Just as with blood counts, there are no hard-and-fast rules about other factors that may preclude a patient from starting interferon therapy. However, some of the other important things that your hepatologist may consider when determining whether interferon is right for you are:

- The level of your disease activity as determined by the liver biopsy. If you have very mild disease, and there are confounding factors such as other medical problems (e.g., heart, kidney, or an auto-immune disease), advanced age, and a history of depression, your doctor may decide to hold off on interferon therapy and monitor you periodically for the time being.
- The results of your hepatitis B e antigen and HBV DNA blood tests, which will show how many copies of the virus are circulating in your blood (more than 200 pg/ml is considered high).
- The results of other laboratory blood tests, including the amount of the protein albumin and of the bile pigment bilirubin.
- Whether or not you have advanced liver disease such as severe cirrhosis. If so, interferon would not be recommended because it could worsen your disease. In this case, your doctor may recommend that you take lamivudine instead.

Once your physician has determined that you are an acceptable candidate for interferon therapy, he or she may check the baseline level of a thyroid hormone called thyroid-stimulating hormone, or TSH, before you begin treatment, because interferon occasionally can cause thyroid dysfunction (see pages 39–40).

How is interferon administered? If your liver specialist gives you the go-ahead to take interferon for your HBV infection, you will be taught to inject yourself with this antiviral medicine "subcutaneously" (that is, just under the skin, rather than deeply into the muscle). At our medical center, we ask patients who are starting interferon treatment to set up an appointment at the learning center so that the staff can show them how to inject themselves with this drug. Patients are asked to bring the medication with them to this appointment so that they can inject themselves.

You will be shown how to cleanse your injection site with alcohol before you give yourself a shot. Make sure that you allow the alcohol to dry completely before the injection; otherwise, the wet alcohol can be very irritating. Injecting into the same area repeatedly can also lead to redness and irritation, so your injection sites should be rotated (for example, if you use your right thigh on Monday for the injection, use your left thigh on Wednesday).

We ask our patients to make sure that someone can accompany them home after their injection class in case they experience side effects.

What are the side effects of interferon therapy? If you are taking interferon, your body may react to it in many different ways. Side effects do not occur in all patients; those that do occur are more severe in some individuals and extremely tolerable in others. Symptoms tend to wax and wane and generally are reversible.

When we have the flu, we feel lousy and achy because our bodies produce small amounts of interferon to fight the flu virus. When you take interferon in drug form, you're giving yourself enormous amounts of this substance, so you may experience fever, a flu-like illness, and body aches (malaise). Other common side effects include loss of appetite, irritability, depression, and hair loss. Usually these side effects are manageable; less than 10 percent of patients stop using interferon because of them.

Now let's discuss the potential side effects of this type of drug therapy and what you can do to minimize them.

Systemic flu-like symptoms. When you're taking interferon, you may experience chills followed by a fever, a headache, and muscle aches. These symptoms generally occur four to six hours after the interferon injection. Their duration is variable, but they usually last a few hours. Fortunately, flu-like symptoms tend to lessen and dissipate after a few weeks of therapy.

Many people take their injections a few hours before bedtime so that they can sleep through this side effect. Taking two extra-strength acetaminophen (Tylenol) capsules or tablets (a total of 1 gram) fifteen minutes before your interferon injection also may help. Be sure to sleep with layers of blankets so that you will be warm enough if you feel chilled and comfortable when your body starts to cool down through sweating.

I also advise my patients to drink plenty of noncaffeinated and non-carbonated fluids every day. To determine how much fluid you should drink daily, divide your weight in half. The resulting number is the number of fluid ounces that you should consume daily. For example, if you weigh 130 pounds, then you should drink approximately 65 ounces, or eight 8-ounce glasses, of fluid. Water, juice, and Gatorade are good choices, as are Jell-O, soups, and popsicles. Make sure that fluids are accessible during the day so that you remember to drink. If you wait until you come home from work at the end of the day to drink all of that fluid, your sleep may be disrupted by frequent trips to the bathroom!

Extra fluids will help to prevent dehydration and the headache and fatigue that may accompany interferon treatment. If you do develop a headache soon after taking this drug, it probably will be short-lived. Although excessive amounts of Tylenol can cause further liver problems (see pages 123–25), you can safely take up to four extra-strength capsules (a total of 2 grams) over a twenty-four-hour period. Aspirin and nonsteroidal anti-inflammatory drugs (such as ibuprofen) also can be used, but they can cause ulcers and internal bleeding and should be avoided if you have cirrhosis or a history of peptic ulcer disease. Ask your doctor which type of pain reliever is most appropriate for you.

Fatigue is usually mild but is occasionally severe. Be sure to get enough rest. You may find that meditation and massage are helpful. I also recommend fifteen minutes of low-level physical exercise (such as walking or swimming) every day to counter fatigue and improve your general feeling of well-being. Although it may be the last thing you want to do because you feel so tired, exercise is one of the best ways to reduce fatigue. Walking and swimming are also good if you're losing weight and muscle mass while you're taking interferon, because they will help to develop the large muscles (quadriceps) in your legs.

If you find that flu-like symptoms strike at odd times (e.g., during the day although you took your interferon the night before), talk to your physician about changing the time of your injection.

Bone marrow suppression. As I mentioned earlier, interferon may suppress your bone marrow so that it cannot produce infection-fighting white blood cells as it should. Frequent blood counts will be taken to determine to what extent interferon is having this effect. If your white blood cell count is low, your risk for infection is high, so it's important to avoid people with colds and other viruses. Wash your hands well and frequently. Check your temperature every day; if it's 101°Fahrenheit or higher, you might have an infection and you should call your physician.

Mental changes. If you have a history of psychiatric disease, your doctor should refer you to a psychiatrist for assessment before you start interferon treatment. If you suffered from depression before you developed HBV infection, you may need to have your antidepressant dosage changed, and your doctor will need to monitor your response to interferon carefully. Even if you haven't had depression or other forms of mental health problems in the past, while you are taking interferon you may experience this mood disorder as a side effect of this drug, as the result of other side effects of this treatment (such as fatigue), or simply as the result of having a long-term illness.

If you haven't had depression before, will you know how to recognize it if you begin to experience it now? According to Lucianna DiMeglio, a nurse who has cared for many patients who have taken interferon, "Depression has many masks," but doctors who suspect that a patient may have depression look for a particular set of symptoms that persist for at least two weeks. Depression usually includes feeling sad and a loss of interest in activities that you used to enjoy, plus three of the following "masks":

- Sleeping too long or not enough
- Over- or undereating
- Excessive guilt or feelings of worthlessness
- Agitation
- Problems concentrating
- Loss of energy
- (Very rarely) thoughts of death

If you have had any of these symptoms before beginning interferon treatment or if they develop while you are undergoing treatment, be sure to tell your physician.

Thyroid problems. Your thyroid, an endocrine gland located at the base of your neck, produces certain hormones that play an important role in regulating your body's metabolic rate. Less than 5 percent of people who are taking interferon develop thyroid abnormalities. If you do, you may need to start taking long-term thyroid hormone replacement therapy, and you will need to see your doctor regularly to monitor the levels of thyroid hormones in your blood.

Eye abnormalities. Interferon treatment also may affect your retina, the sensory membrane that lines the inside of your eyes. As a result, you may develop retinal problems that include bleeding and "cotton-wool spots," or white or gray "floaters." Your risk of developing these complications is higher if you are a diabetic or if you have high blood pressure or a history of eye problems (other than needing eyeglasses). If you fall within this high-risk group, you should have a baseline retinal examination before starting treatment with interferon.

If you develop eye problems while undergoing interferon therapy, your physician can refer you to an ophthalmologist. Serious eye problems related to interferon therapy are very rare.

Miscellaneous side effects. In addition to the various side effects that I've just described, some patients experience hair thinning or hair loss after taking interferon for a while. Although this is an uncommon side effect, it's nevertheless distressing for those who experience it. This condition is usually mild and reversible, and it can be minimized by using gentle hair products and washing your hair every other day rather than daily.

Some people also have restless sleep and dreams and, rarely, vivid and even bizarre nightmares. For those with insomnia, I often prescribe 12.5 to 25 mg daily of a drug called amitriptyline. Adjusting the time or days of your interferon injections also may be helpful. For instance, changing the time of your injection to the morning may alleviate your sleeplessness and the fatigue that may be associated with it.

Good communication with your doctor and health care team is especially important while you are undergoing treatment for HBV infection. You may wish to carry a small notebook to jot down questions for your doctor as they come to mind. Then, when you go to your appointment, you can review these questions with your doctor.

A notebook also can help you keep track of how you are feeling both physically and mentally. A record of the specific side effect that you may be feeling, the time(s) of day when it occurs, and which measures make it better or worse will enable your physician to help you manage your symptoms.

How successful is this drug? The success of your interferon treatment will depend on several variables, including:

1. How long you've had chronic HBV infection. The shorter the duration of your infection, the better your response will be.
2. Where you were born. The response rate may be lower in people who were born in Asia, because in that part of the world transmission of HBV often occurs during birth or early childhood. Hence, if you were born in Asia and you were infected with HBV early in life, you will have had the disease for a relatively long time, and your response to interferon may not be as good as it might be if you were born elsewhere and you acquired the infection later in life.
3. How abnormal the results of your liver enzyme blood tests are. The higher the level of your liver enzymes (ALT and AST), the better your response will be to interferon.
4. Whether or not you also have hepatitis D ("delta") virus (HDV) infection. HDV "piggybacks" onto the hepatitis B virus and can make your illness more severe. We don't know why, but coinfection with the HDV virus can worsen your response to interferon.

How will I know if interferon is working? The ideal goal of treatment for viral hepatitis infections is to eradicate the virus completely from the bloodstream. If this is not possible, an achievable secondary goal is to interrupt the virus's ability to multiply, or replicate. Liver experts generally use three specific blood tests to determine whether or not this viral inhibition is occurring:

1. They look for a decrease in the number of copies of the virus that are circulating in your blood. This drop in viral load will be apparent from a decreased HBV-DNA level.
2. They also may look for a conversion of the HBV e antigen to the e antibody.

3. Finally, hepatologists look for a decrease or normalization in the level of liver enzymes (ALT and AST) in the blood; this decrease may be associated with fewer damaged liver cells (hepatocytes).

Most often, based on the results of these blood tests, your liver specialist will be able to determine whether or not your condition is improving. A repeat liver biopsy usually isn't necessary.

LAMIVUDINE. In addition to interferon, a drug called lamivudine (also called 3TC or Epivir) may be an effective option to treat your chronic HBV infection. Lamivudine has been used for many years for the treatment of AIDS, but it was approved for the treatment of HBV infection only recently. In contrast to interferon, lamivudine is given by mouth, not by injections. It is extremely well tolerated; there are no significant side effects. Recent studies have shown that it can be effective (it works 15 to 20 percent of the time). Then what's the drawback?

The major concern with lamivudine is that in up to one-fourth of patients who take it for one year, the hepatitis B virus becomes resistant to the drug, and we don't know what the long-term consequences of this drug resistance will be. This is such a concern worldwide that many scientists are actively investigating which patients should take lamivudine, how long they should take it, and whether or not it should be combined with other drugs. Some hepatologists—and I am one of them—feel that we need to convene a National Institutes of Health (NIH) consensus conference to frame the right questions regarding HBV and then do the appropriate studies that will shed light on many different aspects of treatment.

As always, talk with your physician about whether this drug is a good choice for you.

NEW DRUGS ON THE HORIZON. Many other medications are being studied extensively for the treatment of chronic HBV infection. These agents, which include famciclovir, gancyclovir, acyclovir, and lobucavir, are being tested in clinical trials throughout the world. Famciclovir, when administered in doses of 500 mg three times per day, has been found to result in significant viral suppression and achievement of normal serum ALT levels even in patients who have severe liver disease and in those who have received a liver transplant. Ongoing studies regarding famciclovir, as well as other agents such as FTC and adefovir dipivoxil, will determine the true place of these medications in the treatment of chronic HBV infection.

Novel vaccines also are being investigated. Although most vaccines are used to prevent infection, these vaccines are being tried for treatment of already established disease.

LIVER TRANSPLANTATION

I want to reassure you that most patients with HBV infection do *not* require a liver transplant. However, if you have "end-stage" liver disease—that is, if your liver is damaged to such an extent that you have cirrhosis with life-threatening complications such as bleeding from ruptured veins in the esophagus, a liver transplant may be a lifesaving treatment option.

In this major operation, liver transplant surgeons replace the patient's entire diseased liver with a healthy liver from a deceased donor. It's also possible to transplant part of a healthy liver from a living donor; the donor's remaining liver and the recipient's "new" liver will regenerate (grow back to its original full size) within a few weeks. Liver transplants are discussed in great detail in chapter 13. For now, though, I'd like to answer the most common questions that my patients with HBV infection tend to ask.

WILL I NEED A LIVER TRANSPLANT? If you have *acute* HBV infection, you have a 99 percent chance of recovering from the acute episode. You would only need a liver transplant if you had fulminant liver failure—that is, if you suddenly developed very severe disease. In this condition, called fulminant hepatitis B, a liver transplant is the only treatment of merit.

If your HBV infection is *chronic* and your disease is not severe, you probably will be given one of two drugs: interferon or lamivudine. However, if you develop cirrhosis or any significant life-threatening complications, a liver transplant may be necessary.

WHAT IS THE SUCCESS RATE FOR LIVER TRANSPLANTATION FOR HBV? The overall survival rate is as high as 80 percent one year after the operation and 65 percent three years after the operation. Patients who have

---

Questions to Ask Your Liver Specialist
if You Have Been Diagnosed with Chronic HBV

- How severe is my HBV infection?
- Am I a candidate for treatment with drug therapy with interferon or lamivudine?
- Are there ongoing drug protocol studies (for new medicines) that I might qualify for? If so, is there a major center in my area that is doing such a study?
- Are there any ramifications for my family? Should the other people in my home be vaccinated?
- Should I stop drinking alcohol?
- Will I need a liver transplant?
- What is my risk of developing liver cancer? If I am at risk, how should I be screened for it?

---

combined HBV and hepatitis D (delta) infection and patients with fulminant HBV infection generally have a better prognosis than patients who simply have chronic HBV.

WHAT ARE THE CHANCES THAT MY HBV INFECTION WILL COME BACK AFTERWARD?
If you have acute HBV infection with fulminant hepatic failure, your risk of disease recurrence after liver transplantation is lower than it is for people who have a liver transplant because of chronic HBV infection. Chapter 13 provides more details about ways to prevent disease recurrence.

HEPATITIS C VIRUS

The *hepatitis C virus (HCV)* used to be called "non-A, non-B hepatitis," because scientists recognized that many cases of what was almost certainly viral hepatitis were caused by something other than the hepatitis A or B virus. Although researchers still haven't figured out how to cultivate this elusive virus reliably in the laboratory, in 1989 Michael Houghton and his colleagues used molecular biological techniques to clone hepatitis C, the agent responsible for 90 percent of non-A, non-B hepatitis in Western countries. At a symposium in early 1999, one investigator presented a model of the impact of HCV infection in the United States by the year 2008. This model predicts that

- the incidence of primary cancer of the liver (also called primary hepatocellular carcinoma, or hepatoma) due to HCV will increase twofold.
- liver-related deaths will increase fourfold.
- the need for liver transplants will increase sixfold.

The resulting health care costs certainly will be staggering! Moreover, the deaths from HCV infection—now an estimated 10,000 deaths per year—may triple or even quadruple in the next ten to twenty years and will surpass by far deaths from HIV infection.

Fortunately, we are getting closer to a "cure" for HCV infection with two currently used drugs: interferon and ribavirin. To learn more about HCV infection, turn to the chapters that follow this one (chapters 4–6). There you will find a complete description of the risk factors, symptoms, and diagnostic tests associated with this viral infection, as well as a discussion of current and future treatment options.

HEPATITIS D VIRUS

Another blood-borne pathogen, the *hepatitis D virus* (also called *delta agent* or *HDV*) was first discovered in 1977 by Dr. Rizzetto and colleagues in Turin, Italy. Like HBV and HCV, the delta virus can cause both acute and chronic hepatitis. The mortality rate from acute delta hepatitis ranges from 2 to 20 percent. The course of chronic delta hepatitis also tends to be more serious than that of chronic HBV and HCV infection.

Delta virus needs to coexist with HBV infection. This interrelationship is very important; long-term studies indicate that approximately 75 percent of people who are infected with chronic delta hepatitis and chronic HBV infection at the same time go on to develop cirrhosis and its complications, which include accumulation of fluid within the abdomen (ascites) and engorged veins called varices in the esophagus (see chapter 9). The incidence of such complications in patients who have chronic HBV infection *without* chronic HDV infection is far lower—25 percent.

Are You at Risk?

Endemic delta virus infection (that is, HDV infection that is prevalent in a particular area) is common in the Middle East, the Mediterranean, Korea, South America, and Romania. In contrast, the incidence of endemic HDV is low in the United States, North Africa, Northern Europe, and China.

Epidemic (or a sudden spread of) delta virus infection usually occurs in isolated populations in underdeveloped areas of the world. For instance, well-defined outbreaks have been documented in the Amazon basin. In these outbreaks, HDV infection (also called Labrea fever in this area) is particularly severe, with the rapid onset of acute liver failure accompanied by altered or depressed consciousness (or fulminant hepatitis) and a downhill, fatal course. The mortality rate for this extreme form of HDV illness, which frequently affects children, approaches 20 percent.

Like hepatitis B and C, which also can be spread by contact with infected blood, hepatitis D afflicts certain high-risk groups, including intravenous drug addicts, hemophiliacs, and homosexual men.

Your doctor should suspect HDV infection and give you appropriate tests to look for it if you have severe acute or chronic HBV infection or fulminant HBV infection, or if you have chronic HBV and you develop worsening liver disease.

Prevention

Delta hepatitis infection is linked inextricably to HBV infection, so its prevention is related closely to the prevention of that virus. I'm hopeful that the widespread (and ideally universal) use of the HBV vaccine will result in the elimination of this virulent pathogen. There is no available vaccine for the hepatitis D virus.

Symptoms

The symptoms of delta hepatitis are practically indistinguishable from those related to any other form of acute and chronic viral hepatitis— although on average they are more severe. Thus, if you are infected with this virus you may have mild jaundice, weakness, and fatigue. You may experience nausea and lose your appetite, and you may feel discomfort in the right upper part of your abdomen, where your liver is located.

If you have both chronic HDV and chronic HBV infection, and these infections have caused cirrhosis, you also may have serious complications of that condition, including a swollen, fluid-filled abdomen (ascites) and swollen, engorged veins called varices in your esophagus. If these varices burst, you may vomit or pass blood rectally. Such bleeding requires immediate medical attention.

Finally, if your HBV infection is accompanied by HDV, you may develop sudden, severe hepatic failure. With fulminant liver failure, toxins such as ammonia accumulate in the body because the liver can no longer clear such poisons from the blood effectively. These toxins can affect the brain and may cause mental changes ranging from mild confusion to coma.

Diagnosis

There are no specific telltale signs for delta infection on physical examination. As with other forms of viral hepatitis, though, if you have HDV infection, your doctor may find that your liver and spleen are enlarged when he or she examines you. With HDV infection, blood tests usually show elevated levels of the liver enzymes alanine transaminase (ALT) and aspartate transaminase (AST). Gastroenterologists and hepatologists routinely check patients with severe, acute fulminant HBV infection and patients with chronic HBV infection for delta infection. Specific blood tests called the HDV antibody test and the HDV-RNA test can confirm the diagnosis.

Treatment

DRUG THERAPY. Unfortunately, there is no proven drug therapy for delta hepatitis. Drugs called corticosteroids will not be helpful if you have this disease. Indeed, steroids will simply cause the virus to multiply further.

One well-designed study showed that interferon, when given for one year, appeared to stop the delta hepatitis virus from multiplying, and resulted in improved levels of liver enzymes (ALT and AST). However, most of the patients experienced a significant clinical relapse when they stopped taking this drug. Whether interferon treatment given for a longer period of time, or larger doses of interferon in combination with lamivudine, will be helpful in abating this disease remains to be determined.

LIVER TRANSPLANTATION. If your HDV infection is severe—that is, if it produces end-stage liver disease with multiple complications or fulminant hepatic failure as I described earlier—your doctor may recommend that you undergo a liver transplant.

Although the idea of such a major procedure may be overwhelming at first, you should be encouraged to know that people with HDV infection have had excellent results with this operation (see chapter 13). In fact, having HDV actually may be beneficial, since HDV appears to inhibit the hepatitis B virus from multiplying. Thus, coinfection with both viruses can lower your risk of disease recurrence. Taking drugs such as interferon or lamivudine after this operation should lower your risk of recurrence even further.

HEPATITIS E VIRUS

Besides hepatitis C, there is another form of non-A, non-B hepatitis. At first it was called *enterically transmitted non-A, non-B* or *waterborne non-A, non-B hepatitis* (because it's usually spread by contaminated water). Now this virus is called *hepatitis E (HEV)*.

Like HAV, HEV infection never leads to chronic liver disease.

Are You at Risk?

In Western countries, HEV is a very rare disorder, and in a sense it's almost always "imported." Most cases of HEV infection occur in India, Pakistan, Nepal, Africa, Mexico, and Central and Southeast Asia. Rare, sporadic cases also have been reported among travelers visiting regions where this virus is endemic.

One of the worst recorded outbreaks of HEV infection occurred in Delhi, India, in the winter of 1955–56. Heavy rains led to the flooding of the Yamuna River, and recession of the floodwaters led to a backup of a large open drain and subsequent contamination of the water supply. Despite immediate and extensive chlorination of the water, almost 30,000 people were afflicted with HEV. Since then, in several different parts of the world there have been similar attacks in which thousands of individuals have been affected.

The HEV virus tends to affect people in the fifteen- to forty-year age group, and it is associated with a high (10 to 20 percent) fatality rate among pregnant women who are infected.

Prevention

The best way to protect yourself from this type of viral hepatitis is to avoid potentially contaminated food and water. No vaccine is currently available.

Symptoms

The symptoms of HEV infection are similar to those seen in patients with acute HAV or HBV: they include fever, malaise, a distaste for tobacco, loss of appetite, and jaundice.

Diagnosis

If you have HEV infection, your physician may find that you have an enlarged liver and spleen and that you have jaundice.

The only way to confirm the diagnosis of HEV infection is through a blood test that can be performed at the U.S. Centers for Disease Control (CDC) or in some special laboratories. Thus, if your physician suspected that you may have HEV, she would have to send a sample of your blood to the CDC or to one of these labs to screen for the virus.

Treatment

There is no proven medicine to counteract HEV infection. If you are infected with this virus, your doctor most likely will recommend that you rest and drink a lot of fluids. Most people recover fully on their own without any form of treatment. If your infection is more severe, bed rest and intravenous fluids may be required. In patients with fulminant hepatic failure, the only treatment is liver transplantation.

WHY ISN'T THERE A "HEPATITIS F" VIRUS?

In 1991 and 1992, some Japanese investigators described preliminary evidence of a hepatitis virus that they designated *hepatitis F virus*. This discovery has not been borne out in subsequent studies. As Harvey Alter, an eminent hepatologist at the CDC, recently said, "The hepatitis F virus has simply gotten flushed down the toilet."

HEPATITIS G VIRUS

The *hepatitis G virus (HGV)* may or may not cause bona fide liver disease in humans. It may be found in people who have unexplained acute liver failure accompanied by mental confusion and even coma ("acute fulminant hepatitis"); chronic hepatitis that is presumed to be viral, but is not caused by the hepatitis B, C, or D viruses; cirrhosis for which there is no known cause; and a form of liver cancer called primary hepatocellular carcinoma.

Blood banks that do a polymerase chain reaction (PCR) test to look for the RNA of this virus have found that HGV also is present among healthy blood donors in the United States. Does that mean that you're at great risk of contracting viral hepatitis if you receive donated blood? Not at all. In fact, the incidence of posttransfusion hepatitis has dropped from 1 in 20 just a few decades ago to an estimated 1 in 100,000 currently—in spite of the continued use of donor blood that is positive for HGV. Thus, HGV does not appear to be a bona fide factor in causing posttransfusion hepatitis.

Even more importantly, scientists do not think that the hepatitis G virus causes liver disease in any meaningful fashion. Several dozen studies have shown that people who have HCV infection alone and people who have both HCV and HGV infection at the same time have an identical clinical picture. In other words, their liver function test results, liver biopsy results, response to medications like interferon, and incidence of disease recurrence after liver transplantation are all the same. HGV doesn't appear to worsen even already-existing liver disease.

TABLE 3-1

The Alphabet Soup of Viral Hepatitis

Type of virus	New infections/year	Transmission	Causes acute liver disease	Causes chronic liver disease	Risk of cirrhosis and cancer of the liver (hepatoma)	Diagnosis (blood tests)	Vaccine available?	Treatment*
Hepatitis A	Approx. 200,000	Via contaminated food or water and via fecal contamination	Yes	No	None	*Acute HAV:* IgM anti-HAV positive. *Past infection and recovery:* IgG anti-HAV positive	Yes	*For acute HAV:* bed rest, rarely steroids (for cholestatic HAV infection)
Hepatitis B	150,000–300,000	Via contact with infected blood (e.g., from unsterilized needles, sex with an infected person, transmission from infected mothers to newborns) (however, in the U.S. and many other countries pregnant women are screened and all infants are immunized at birth)	Yes	Yes	Risk of cirrhosis; risk of hepatoma	*Acute HBV:* IgM anti-HBc; hepatitis B surface antigen (HBsAg) usually positive. *Chronic HBV:* HBsAg positive, IgG anti-HBc positive	Yes	Interferon, lamivudine

(continued)

TABLE 3-1 (continued)

Type of virus	New infections/year	Transmission	Causes acute liver disease	Causes chronic liver disease	Risk of cirrhosis and cancer of the liver (hepatoma)	Diagnosis (blood tests)	Vaccine available?	Treatment*
Hepatitis C	30,000	Via contact with infected blood (e.g., from unsterilized needles, receipt of blood or blood products, especially before 1992, sex with an infected person, and from mothers to newborns) (see chapter 4)	Yes	Yes	Risk of both cirrhosis and hepatoma	*Acute HCV:* HCV-RNA-PCR positive; HCV antibody positive, but may be negative early in the illness. *Chronic HCV:* HCV-RNA-PCR positive. HCV antibody positive	No	Interferon; interferon-ribavirin combination therapy (Rebetron) (see chapter 6)
Hepatitis D	5,000	Persons with hepatitis B may contract hepatitis D via contact with infected blood (e.g., unsterilized needles, sex with an infected person)	Yes	Yes	Risk of both cirrhosis and hepatoma	Hepatitis delta antibody positive; HDV-RNA-PCR positive	No	No proven effective treatment. Patients respond to interferon during treatment, but there is an extremely high rate of relapse following cessation of treatment

TABLE 3-1 (continued)

Type of virus	New infections/year	Transmission	Causes acute liver disease	Causes chronic liver disease	Risk of cirrhosis and cancer of the liver (hepatoma)	Diagnosis (blood tests)	Vaccine available?	Treatment*
Hepatitis E	Rare in the U.S.	Contaminated water in certain parts of the world such as Mexico, India, Pakistan, Nepal, Somalia, Algeria, Russia. In the U.S., HEV is only seen in travelers to those parts of the world or visitors from those countries	Yes	No	None	Blood test not routinely available, but can be requested from CDC	No	Supportive treatment similar to that for HAV

*If the hepatitis is fulminant (if it comes on suddenly with great severity leading to "liver failure") due to any of these viruses, the only proven treatment is liver transplantation.

TTV Virus

Many people may be infected with a DNA virus called transfusion-transmitted virus (TTV), which was discovered in 1998. Although this virus has been detected in roughly 1 percent of blood donors in the United States, 2 percent of blood donors in the United Kingdom, and 12 percent of blood donors in Japan, it's unclear whether TTV causes significant liver disease. As with the hepatitis G virus, scientists are exploring what role, if any, it may play in both acute and chronic liver disease.

4

....

Hepatitis C:
Are You at Risk?

*About ten years ago I experienced some rectal bleeding that
turned out to be a sign of colon cancer. I had an operation, and
now I seem to be a cancer survivor, because I've had three
colonoscopy exams since then and they've been completely
normal. I guess I'm lucky because they caught my cancer at an
early stage.*

*However, I did receive a couple of units of blood during my
operation, and I just received a letter from the hospital saying
that I have a low chance of having acquired hepatitis C from that
blood. I saw my doctor, and he said not to be alarmed—he can
test me, and if I do have hepatitis C, he'll send me to a specialist.
Apparently there are treatments available.*

—MIGUEL SANCHEZ, age fifty-nine

Hepatitis C is a common viral infection that occurs worldwide
and affects an estimated 4 million Americans. Although more Americans
have the hepatitis C virus (HCV) than the human immunodeficiency
virus (HIV, the virus that causes AIDS), an estimated one-fourth to one-
third of individuals with chronic HCV don't even know that they are
infected!

This lack of knowledge is a serious matter, because HCV infection,
when it progresses, does so stealthily over decades, so that by the time

many people first come to clinical attention they already may have advanced liver disease such as distortion of the liver because of severe scarring (cirrhosis; see chapter 9).

According to the U.S. Centers for Disease Control (CDC), 10,000 people die of hepatitis C each year, and annual deaths from this virus are expected to double or triple by the year 2010. Hence, this disease has been called "the silent epidemic" and "the shadow epidemic," and the hepatitis C virus has been dubbed "a wolf in sheep's clothing."

What is hepatitis C? Are you at risk for acquiring this infection? As I noted in chapter 3, the word *hepatitis* means "inflammation of the liver." Hepatitis C infection is inflammation of the liver that is caused by the hepatitis C virus. It's commonly spread directly from one person to another via infected blood or indirectly, via contaminated needles. I'll talk about other modes of transmission a little later in this chapter.

ACUTE VS. CHRONIC HCV INFECTION

If you have hepatitis C infection you may have either an *acute* or *chronic* (long-term) case of the disease. Although people of all ages can be infected with the hepatitis C virus, most people with acute HCV infection are between the ages of twenty and thirty-nine years, and most people with chronic HCV infection are between the ages of thirty and forty-nine years. Experts expect the number of HCV-related deaths to jump significantly in the next twenty years because many infected people will be reaching the ages at which serious complications of long-term liver disease generally occur.

In the United States, acute HCV infections account for one-fifth of all cases of acute hepatitis. There are approximately 30,000 new acute HCV infections each year, of which only about 25 percent are diagnosed. A recent report by the CDC indicates that African Americans and whites have a similar reported incidence of acute disease; Hispanics have higher rates of acute infection. In contrast, chronic HCV infection is more common among African Americans than whites.

Acute Infection

As you read in chapter 3, acute hepatitis means that the liver has been injured recently and is severely inflamed. If you have an acute case of HCV infection, you probably will have flu-like symptoms and perhaps jaundice. I'll talk more about the symptoms and diagnosis of acute infection in the next chapter.

If you have acute hepatitis C and are fortunate enough not to develop chronic (long-term) HCV infection, you may have had either a mild or a severe episode of the disease, but in either case you will go on to recover with no significant adverse effects. Of all patients who get acute hepatitis C infection, only 20 percent or so are this lucky.

Chronic Infection

Chronic, or long-lasting, infection means that you've had HCV for more than six months. Of those individuals who acquire acute HCV infection, 80 percent go on to become chronically infected. If you do have chronic HCV, you probably will be saddled with lifelong infection. Although virtually no one recovers spontaneously (on their own) from chronic HCV infection, you may have only a mild case of the disease for many decades.

Your prognosis is best if you are a woman, if you do not drink alcohol, and if you acquired your hepatitis infection before the age of thirty-five years. If this is the case, you may never develop cirrhosis (severe scarring and distortion of the liver that can cause serious and even life-threatening complications), or it may take forty to eighty years to develop cirrhosis. In contrast, if you are a man, if you drink more than 50 grams of alcohol (or four drinks)* per day, and if you became infected with HCV after the age of forty-five years, your prognosis is not as good; you may develop cirrhosis within ten to twelve years.

HOW DOES A PERSON GET HEPATITIS C?

The hepatitis C virus is a blood-borne pathogen, and your risk of being infected with it is highest if you have ever used an unsterilized needle

---

*One standard drink is 6 ounces of wine, 12 ounces of beer, or 1.5 ounces of 90-proof spirits.

while taking intravenous drugs or if you received blood or blood products (such as clotting factors, platelet transfusions, or a certain brand of gamma globulin—see page 59) before 1992, when good screening measures for this virus became available. (As I'll explain a bit later on, today the risk of acquiring HCV from blood products is negligible.)

Intravenous Drug Abuse

A major reason for the spread of hepatitis C is that this virus is blood-borne, and drug users often share needles. In fact, intravenous drug abuse is responsible for 60 percent of all new HCV infections.

According to the U.S. Centers for Disease Control, the rate of HCV infection among intravenous drug users is four times higher than the rate of HIV infection. Half of all drug addicts become infected within the first six months of starting this dangerous habit, and as many as 75 percent are infected by the end of the first year! Because of their high rate of drug abuse, there is also a high incidence of chronic HCV infection among prisoners.

Although heavy drug abusers appear to have the greatest risk, if you used intravenous drugs even just "a couple of times" decades ago, you may have acquired HCV. Indeed, my patients are shocked to learn that something they experimented with in a most casual fashion twenty or twenty-five years ago could now be affecting their health or be a reason for life insurance denial.

Receipt of Blood or Blood Products

Although the risk of acquiring HCV infection from intravenous drug injection remains high, the risk of acquiring this virus from the transfusion of blood or blood products has declined dramatically in the last couple of decades. In the 1960s, approximately one-third of patients who received blood transfusions in the United States became infected with HCV. By the late 1970s and early 1980s, though, only 5 percent of such people acquired HCV infection. Hemophiliacs, patients on long-term dialysis, those who had severe trauma or major abdominal surgery (like Miguel, the patient at the beginning of this chapter), and those who had a coronary artery bypass graft or other kinds of cardiac surgery had a particularly high risk of contracting hepatitis C because they often required multiple blood transfusions. They also may have received fresh frozen plasma, which often is pooled from several donors.

In the early 1990s, several hundred people became infected with HCV after using an intravenous immune globulin product called Gammagard. They had been given this blood product between March 1993 and February 1994. In February 1994 the manufacturer, Baxter Healthcare Corporation, and the American Red Cross (which had distributed this product under the name Polygam) recalled this HCV-contaminated lot of immune globulin and notified the people who had received it.

As unfortunate as this incident was, you should know that all *current* lots of gamma globulin are deemed to be free of the virus, and if you are receiving this blood product now, you should feel secure about its safety. Likewise, if you or someone you love currently requires blood transfusions, you should feel confident that the risk of contracting hepatitis C from donor blood is now exceedingly low—about 1 in 100,000 units of blood transfused. This remarkable decline in risk has come about only recently with the discovery of hepatitis C and the mandatory testing of each unit of donor blood for the HCV antibody (a marker of potential infection).

Unfortunately, such careful screening methods were not available until 1992. In 1990 blood banks began trying to exclude transmission of this virus *indirectly* by using so-called surrogate marker tests. That is, if the donor's blood revealed an elevated level of a liver enzyme called alanine transaminase (ALT) or was positive for the hepatitis B core antibody, there was a chance that this donor was in fact infected with hepatitis C, and that the use of his blood might lead to the transmission of HCV. Every single unit of blood was tested, and if the ALT was elevated or the HBV core antibody was positive, the blood was excluded from the blood supply. These tests were clearly helpful in decreasing the spread of what was then called non-A, non-B hepatitis (now hepatitis C). However, these measures did not screen *directly* for the hepatitis C virus, and hence the blood supply was still at a significant risk for contamination until the more accurate screening test for the actual hepatitis C virus became available in 1992. These days, blood banks are beginning to use even more precise molecular techniques to detect viruses such as HCV and HIV, the virus that causes AIDS. Eventually such techniques may eradicate these viruses from the blood supply for good.

Table 4-1 illustrates the long-term potential health risks for people who received blood transfusions before each unit of blood was screened for the HCV antibody.

You may be wondering why, with the availability of these sensitive and effective tests for hepatitis C, a risk still exists, however small, of transmission of the virus through the blood supply. This risk remains because a blood donor who recently was exposed to hepatitis C could have the virus circulating in his or her bloodstream, but may feel perfectly healthy and may donate blood. The blood would be accepted and considered safe for transfusion purposes because the individual is in a "window period" when antibodies are not yet detectable; hence the commonly performed blood test for hepatitis C would be negative (i.e., would not reveal the virus).

The good news is that the Red Cross, which oversees almost half of the U.S. blood supply, recently moved to close this window period by approving a solvent detergent "cleaner" for blood plasma. This treatment inactivates the viruses that cause AIDS, hepatitis B, and hepatitis C, but does not harm the important proteins that plasma can provide. With the continued development of such solutions, HCV likely will be eradicated completely from the national blood supply in our lifetime.

TABLE 4-1

Risk of Acquiring HCV from Blood Transfusions Prior to 1992

3 million people received blood transfusions each year in the United States
⇩
5 percent, or 150,000 people, developed acute HCV
⇩
75 percent, or 112,500, of those people who developed acute HCV went on to develop chronic HCV
⇩
An estimated 25 percent of chronically infected people, or 28,000, will develop cirrhosis (generally after twenty years)
⇩
1–4 percent of people, or 280–1,120, with cirrhosis will develop liver cancer each year.

Organ Transplants

For the reasons I've just described, it's also theoretically possible—though rare in this age of careful screening—to contract hepatitis C if you receive an organ transplant and the organ donor was infected with the virus. As with the receipt of blood products, your risk of contracting HCV from a donor organ would have been much higher a decade ago.

Tattooing, Body Piercing, and Acupuncture

Any type of needle that has been used by a person with HCV can infect another person if it is used again without being sterilized properly. The increasingly popular practices of tattooing, body piercing, and acupuncture thus present certain risks of disease transmission, although how often such transmission occurs is unknown.

Tattooing is practiced in most cultures all over the world. In the United States, people from all walks of life—including students, gang members, prisoners, members of the military, famous athletes, and Hollywood celebrities—often have visible tattoos decorating their bodies. At a recent lecture that I gave to high school students in Biloxi, Mississippi, I asked how many students had a tattoo or were seriously contemplating getting one. Three-quarters of the young people in the auditorium raised their hands!

If you get a tattoo, though, you may leave the tattoo parlor with more than a colorful design on your skin—you also may have acquired either the hepatitis B or hepatitis C virus. That's because breaks in the skin and bleeding may occur during the tattooing process, and sterilization techniques at some tattoo parlors may be inadequate. For the same reason, another increasingly common practice—body piercing—may pose a risk, especially if the implements used are not sterilized properly and if they are used by many individuals. Similarly, acupuncture may be risky because *any* sharp instruments that are used in or on your body may transmit HCV. Therefore, if you undergo any procedure involving needles, make sure that the practitioner is using sterilized or disposable needles.

Sex

How often does sexual transmission of hepatitis C occur? This question is asked of me almost every day by patients, students, and colleagues in medicine.

Female prostitutes, gay men with multiple sexual partners, and individuals seen in sexually transmitted disease clinics do have a higher incidence of hepatitis C than the rest of the population. You might be tempted, then, to conclude that hepatitis C is sexually transmitted. However, although I have seen several hundred patients with chronic HCV infection in my years of clinical practice, less than 5 percent of them have family members who also are infected with the virus. Furthermore, in a study done a few years ago, investigators used the sensitive polymerase chain reaction (PCR) test to examine semen and saliva specimens from about a dozen men with chronic hepatitis C. Not a single sample was positive for this virus.

Thus, although sexual transmission can occur, it does so infrequently, especially within monogamous relationships. If you have HCV and you have been with a partner for twenty or thirty years (and your partner is tested and is found to be negative for hepatitis C), you don't necessarily have to change your sexual practices. As a precaution, don't have sex during your (or your partner's) menstrual period, and if you're infected, always be sure to cover any open cuts or wounds that you may have. If you have hepatitis C and are just starting a sexual relationship, you may wish to use condoms to have protected sex.

And what should you do if you're sexually involved with someone who has HCV infection? I would advise you to be tested the next time you visit your internist, but you don't have to panic and see someone right away. If you're in a long-term relationship with this partner, there is a *small* risk that you may become infected with HCV over the next decade or so, and thus you may want to be tested for the virus regularly—every two years or so.

Nonsexual Transmission of HCV in Your Home

If you are infected with HCV or if you share your life with someone who is, it's very important to be aware of the facts regarding HCV transmission. I've had the sad experience of seeing some of my patients being ostracized or rejected by family members after a diagnosis of chronic hepatitis C was made. Occasionally there is misunderstanding and mistrust, and some wonderful and harmonious family relations that have existed for years are destroyed unnecessarily because of ignorance and fear. People may erroneously think that a person who is infected with HCV is a drug addict or has or at one time led a promiscuous lifestyle.

A patient of mine who was diagnosed with hepatitis C and shared this information with her family was devastated when her daughter prohibited her from hugging or cuddling her granddaughter. Another patient was literally told to leave his home by his wife, who completely shunned him for more than a year. She felt that he had a "dirty disease" and that he also might be infected with the AIDS virus—when in reality he had no risk factors for AIDS and probably had acquired HCV infection from a blood transfusion many, many years ago.

It's extremely unlikely that hepatitis C is transmitted casually, so it's perfectly appropriate to hug, kiss, share food (like popcorn or cotton candy), and use common utensils. The only "household" precautions that you should be aware of involve the use of any instruments that may serve as conduits of infected blood—thus, you should *not* share toothbrushes, razor blades, or nail clippers.

Transmission from a Mother to Her Newborn

I got married two years ago, and my husband and I want to start a family. I thought it would be a good idea for me to finally, at the age of twenty-nine, be a little more responsible about my health. So I made an appointment to see my primary care doctor.

She told me that everything looked normal and that she would get back to me about the results of the blood tests that she took. A few days later I got a phone call from her saying that I may have a liver problem. She wanted me to come in to repeat the tests.

I did that, and found out that I have hepatitis C! When I went to see the liver specialist I had so many questions: What does this mean? Can I have a baby? If I do, can I give this virus to my child? Will it be safe to breastfeed?

If, like this patient of mine, you are infected with HCV and you are thinking of having a child (or are already pregnant), you may wonder if you can pass this virus along to your baby. The answer is that you may transmit the virus to your newborn, but the risk is on the low side—5 percent. A more positive way to look at this is to say that there is a 95 percent chance that your baby will *not* be infected. (However, your risk of transmitting HCV doubles if you also have HIV infection; if this is the case, you should talk with your doctor about the risks associated with having these two coexisting infections.)

Given the relatively low risk of passing HCV on to your infant, if you are pregnant or planning to conceive, you should not let the presence of the virus interfere with your decision to have a family. Your baby can be tested for HCV when he is a few months old using a sensitive polymerase chain reaction (PCR) test. If he is found to have the virus, a pediatric gastroenterologist or hepatologist will be able to advise you about what should be done.

Note that if an HCV antibody test (rather than a PCR test) is used to screen your child for the virus, the result may be positive for the first few months after your baby's birth simply because the HCV antibody has been transmitted through the placenta. The presence of this antibody does not necessarily mean that your infant is infected. Hence, if the antibody test is going to be used, it should be done when your baby is approximately eighteen months old.

Lastly, if you have hepatitis C you can breast-feed if you wish to do so; there is no evidence that the virus is transmitted via breast-feeding.

Cocaine Snorting

In my practice I've seen many individuals with chronic HCV infection in whom the only identifiable risk factor is cocaine snorting.

Like contaminated needles that sometimes are used for the injection of intravenous drugs, straws that may be used for snorting cocaine can serve as conduits of infected droplets of blood. There is a high incidence of nosebleeds among people who snort cocaine, and snorting devices are often shared, so these devices can easily be contaminated with hepatitis C, and the virus can spread from one individual to another.

Again, you don't have to be an everyday drug user to become infected with HCV. Even if you only used cocaine a couple of times many years ago, there is a possibility that you may have been infected in this manner, and you should be tested for this virus.

Accidental Needle Punctures

If you're a health care worker, you have a low risk (less than a 10 percent chance) of acquiring hepatitis C if you accidentally stick yourself with a contaminated needle.

In the next two chapters, which describe the symptoms, diagnosis, and treatment of hepatitis C, I'll talk about which tests can be done to look for potential infection after such an accident, and how you can be treated if infection has occurred.

5

. . . .

Hepatitis C:
Symptoms and Diagnosis

Regardless of whether you acquired your chronic hepatitis C virus (HCV) infection from a blood transfusion or at a tattoo parlor, it's entirely possible that you will have no symptoms at all. Very often my patients are completely taken by surprise when I tell them the diagnosis, and they say, "But, Dr. Chopra, I feel fine! How could I possibly have an infection affecting my liver?" Usually I tell such patients to think about the many diseases that do not cause noticeable symptoms, yet still may cause significant bodily harm. For instance, you can have a common malady like high blood pressure (hypertension) without knowing it, yet this condition can lead to serious complications unless it's diagnosed and treated.

Not everyone with HCV is completely asymptomatic, though. If you have this infection you may experience mild to debilitating fatigue; discomfort in the upper right side of your abdomen, beneath your rib cage; itchy skin; and symptoms related to other conditions that may coexist with HCV infection. I'll talk about these symptoms a little later on. Any of these symptoms may have a dramatic effect on your work and personal life, but as disruptive and even frightening as they may be, it's important to remember that there is *no* correlation between the severity of your symptoms and the severity of your liver disease (as determined by a liver biopsy).

You may have virtually no symptoms and may play tennis, run marathons, work sixty hours a week, and so forth, yet discover that you have a fairly advanced form of liver disease such as cirrhosis. Or you may have debilitating fatigue yet turn out to have mild disease when the liver cells from your liver biopsy are examined under a microscope.

WHAT ARE THE SYMPTOMS OF HCV?

FATIGUE

The fatigue that you may experience with chronic HCV infection can be quite episodic. You may feel well for many days and even exercise vigorously, and then suddenly, out of the blue, find it difficult even to crawl out of bed.

Why hepatitis C does this is not clear. In my experience, other liver disorders (including hepatitis infections that are caused by other viruses—for example, chronic HBV infection) do not seem to affect people in this way.

ABDOMINAL PAIN

Regardless of whether or not you have fatigue, you may feel discomfort or pain in the right side of your abdomen, near your liver, which is located directly beneath your rib cage. Again, this pain—which can occur sporadically for no apparent reason—does not necessarily mean that your liver disease is severe. Under the microscope, your liver tissue (procured most often by doing a liver biopsy) may show only mild disease—and this is really what matters most—even if your symptoms are quite debilitating.

SYMPTOMS OF ESSENTIAL MIXED CRYOGLOBULINEMIA SYNDROME

Numbness and tingling, painful joints, and raised red dots on your legs also can occur with chronic hepatitis C. This constellation of symptoms, which may be accompanied by kidney problems, is known as essential mixed cryoglobulinemia syndrome. Cryoglobulin is a form of protein that commonly circulates in the blood of people with chronic HCV infection, but less than 5 percent of infected people have clinically significant problems related to this condition.

SYMPTOMS OF PORPHYRIA CUTANEA TARDA

Another syndrome that sometimes goes hand in hand with HCV is called porphyria cutanea tarda. This condition, which literally means "purple skin," causes symptoms ranging from minor lesions to severe scarring on sun-exposed areas of the body. This syndrome has been linked to high levels of iron in the liver, so if you have porphyria cutanea tarda, you may be a candidate for iron reduction therapy, or phlebotomy. Phlebotomy is described in more detail in the next chapter (chapter 6).

SYMPTOMS OF FIBROMYALGIA

There also may be a weak association between HCV infection and fibromyalgia, a syndrome that causes fatigue and increased sensitivity to pain in certain muscles, joints, ligaments, and tendons; these areas are called "tender points." Researchers are still exploring what fibromyalgia really is and whether and how the hepatitis C virus contributes to this syndrome.

SYMPTOMS OF CIRRHOSIS

Twenty years after they become infected with HCV, an estimated 25 percent of patients will develop liver scarring, or cirrhosis. Although fatigue and the other symptoms of HCV infection that I have mentioned thus far can affect your life considerably, it's cirrhosis that can put you at risk for liver cancer and other serious, life-threatening complications.

If you've had HCV infection for decades without knowing it, and your first symptoms of this disease are related to cirrhosis, you may experience a variety of expressions of this illness, including fatigue, nausea, and loss of appetite and weight. You also may have itchy skin, jaundice (a yellowish cast to your skin and the whites of your eyes), or increased sensitivity to drugs. If your cirrhosis already is fairly advanced, your ovulation cycle may be disrupted if you are a woman; or, if you are a man, your breasts may get bigger or your testes may get smaller. Finally, if your symptoms are related to complications of cirrhosis, you may have shortness of breath, a tendency to bruise or bleed easily, a swollen, fluid-filled abdomen (this condition is called ascites), or bleeding from ruptured veins, or varices, in your esophagus. The diagnosis and treatment of these serious complications are described in chapter 9.

HOW DOES HCV INFECTION COME TO LIGHT?

When I saw a sign about a blood drive at work, I thought I'd be altruistic and I went to donate. Not long after that, I received a letter from the blood bank that was sponsoring the drive. I was devastated to find out that I might have hepatitis C!

My doctor said that hepatitis C can be spread by intravenous drug use. Well, I may have shared some needles when I was doing drugs twenty years ago, but how could that give me hepatitis C all these years later? And if I do have it, how could I have had it for two decades without knowing?

If there's a chance that you could be infected with HCV, and you don't have any of the symptoms that I've just described, how would you find out that you have the virus?

Like my patient who found out through a blood drive at his office, you may learn about your exposure to the virus almost by happenstance. You may donate blood and then be informed that your blood tested positive for hepatitis C. Also, if you've received blood or blood products, you could receive a letter from a blood bank or the Red Cross that says that sometime before 1992 you were given blood from a donor who was later found to have hepatitis C. The letter would encourage you to see a doctor and be tested for the virus. A while ago, a program was instituted for blood banks to notify the estimated 300,000 individuals who may have received infected blood from transfusions between 1988 and 1992.

Even if you haven't received such a letter, you may seek medical advice on your own because you've read about the hepatitis C epidemic in a newspaper or magazine article or heard about the virus through a friend or acquaintance, and you may recognize that you have a risk factor such as past or current intravenous drug use. You also may want to be tested because a relative or a sexual partner has the virus.

WHAT YOUR DOCTOR MAY FIND

Even if you have no symptoms of HCV infection, when your doctor is examining you, he or she may notice that your liver or spleen is enlarged or that you have other signs of chronic liver disease, such as red palms and spiderlike red blotches on the skin or tenderness in the upper right part of your abdomen, below your rib cage.

Your physician also may order a battery of blood tests that include liver function tests, or LFTs, as part of a comprehensive medical, insurance, or employment examination. Or, during a routine checkup, she may notice that you have a tattoo, or know that you have used (or still use) intravenous drugs, and she may then go on to simply check your LFTs or look for the various hepatitis viruses by means of other special blood tests. If your primary care physician discovers that you have hepatitis C, she may refer you to a specialist in diseases of the digestive tract (gastroenterologist) or a liver specialist (hepatologist) for evaluation and possible treatment. Since these are two rapidly changing fields, I would encourage you to find an experienced and compassionate specialist who is well versed about the nuances of hepatitis C and the latest treatments that are available for it.

If you go to see such a specialist, it would be helpful for you to take along a trusted friend or your spouse (or, if you are a young adult, a parent) with you. He can accompany you to the doctor's office either for the initial visit or after your physician has taken a detailed history and given you a physical examination. Either way, it will be important for both of you to be present to discuss what a diagnosis of chronic HCV infection will mean for your lives.

BLOOD TESTS

Now let's take a closer look at the different kinds of blood tests that your doctor or specialist may use to confirm the diagnosis of HCV infection, to measure the amount of HCV that is circulating in your bloodstream, and to determine which strain of the virus you have. These tests include HCV antibody tests; the HCV-RNA-PCR test; and genotyping.

HCV Antibody Tests

An antibody is a special type of protein that is called into action by other substances (called antigens) as part of your body's immune response to invaders such as viruses. The two kinds of tests that may be used to look for antibodies to HCV in your blood are the ELISA and RIBA tests.

ELISA TESTS. The first enzyme-linked immunosorbent assay (or ELISA I) test became available shortly after the discovery of hepatitis C in 1989. However, quite often people who did not have hepatitis C showed a positive antibody for the virus when they took this test (this is called a false-positive result). More sophisticated tests to look for the virus in such individuals were negative—that is, they did not detect the virus.

In 1993, a more sensitive test called the ELISA II test was developed, and more recently an ELISA III test has been introduced. Although these tests are better than the ELISA I test, getting a positive result still does not necessarily mean that you are actually infected with HCV.

RIBA TEST. Another test that doctors have used to test for HCV in recent years is called the recombinant immunoblast assay (RIBA). If a sample of your blood shows a reaction to two or more hepatitis C antigens, the test is considered positive (that is, there is a good chance that you are indeed infected with the virus). The downside of this test is that it doesn't indicate whether your HCV infection has resolved or is currently active in your blood. Thus, I currently find little use for it.

HCV-RNA-PCR Test

Although the hepatitis C antibody tests (ELISA II or III and RIBA) are quite accurate, they are not 100 percent foolproof. In addition to the risk of a false-positive result, there is a chance that these tests may not be positive even if you have bona fide chronic HCV infection and the hepatitis C virus is circulating in your body. However, if the antibody test result is positive, the result could mean two very different things: you may currently be infected with HCV, or you may have been infected a long time ago and been lucky enough to fight off the virus. The antibody to HCV can be quite durable and may linger in your bloodstream for many years.

The only definitive way to measure the amount of HCV that may be circulating in your bloodstream and to differentiate between past infection and current infection is to do a much more specific test. Although this particular test is very informative, its name is quite unwieldy: it's called the hepatitis C virus RNA polymerase chain reaction test (or HCV-RNA-PCR, or simply PCR test or RNA test for short!).

The diagnosis of HCV infection carries with it all kinds of ramifications, so I feel that it's imperative that doctors confirm an ELISA or RIBA test result by performing an RNA test. With this much more sensitive test, which is available in many commercial laboratories and research laboratories in academic centers, one can detect even a few hundred copies of the hepatitis C virus circulating in your bloodstream. Like many hepatologists, I skip the "confirmatory" antibody test (the RIBA test) altogether, and simply use the RNA test to verify that a person has hepatitis C.

This test is also useful for health care workers who have accidentally stuck themselves with an HCV-contaminated needle. If this happens to you, the best way to ascertain if you are going to come down with hepatitis C is to have an HCV-RNA blood test two weeks after the accident and then again six to eight weeks later.

You may be wondering what kind of result you might expect with an HCV-RNA test. I see a great deal of variability in these test results among my many patients. A short while ago, for instance, in the same afternoon I saw six consecutive patients in whom hepatitis C had been recently diagnosed. One of them had 242,000 copies of the virus per milliliter (ml) of blood; another had 6.72 million copies per ml; and the other four patients had levels in between these two values.

In general, less than 2 million copies of the virus per milliliter of blood is considered to be a low level—and a low level is good, because it means that you may respond better to treatment with a drug regimen consisting of interferon and ribavirin than you would if you had a high level.

Genotyping

In addition to the antibody and HCV-RNA-PCR tests, if you've been diagnosed with HCV your physician may have you get another blood test to determine which genotype of the virus you have. This is because there is more than one genetic strain, or genotype, of the hepatitis C virus. The virus that's affecting you is one member (genotype) of a whole family of viruses. Each genotype in turn has different subtypes, which are referred to as 1A, 1B, and so on. Scientists have identified at least six distinct genotypes and numerous subtypes of the hepatitis C virus.

Different subtypes of HCV predominate in different parts of the world. Approximately 70 percent of people who are infected with this virus in the United States are infected with genotype 1A or 1B. Your genotype is relevant because if you have a genotype *other* than 1A or 1B (for example, genotype 2 or 3), you have a better chance of achieving a sustained response to interferon and ribavirin (see pages 91–92). Also, the duration of treatment with this regimen could be shorter.

Recent studies suggest that the duration of combination interferon and ribavirin treatment should be dictated by the patient's genotype. That's because in people with genotype 1, forty-eight weeks of treatment results in a greater sustained response rate than twenty-four weeks of treatment. In contrast, for those with other genotypes (2 or 3), we have found that twenty-four weeks of treatment are just as effective as forty-eight weeks. Your specialist should be aware of the latest recommendations regarding the relationship of your genotype to the best treatment option for you.

Genotyping is done routinely in all clinical research studies regarding hepatitis C and is available through several U.S. commercial laboratories.

Laboratory Tests of Liver Function

In addition to the important HCV-RNA-PCR test to actually measure the amount of virus circulating in your blood, your doctor will check liver enzymes and liver function tests (LFTs); these tests make up your liver profile.

LIVER ENZYMES. Two commonly performed tests are the alanine transaminase (ALT; also called serum glutamic pyruvic transaminase, or SGPT) and aspartate transaminase (AST; also called serum glutamic oxaloacetic transaminase, or SGOT). You'll hear these tests most often referred to simply as "ALT and AST" or "liver enzymes." ALT and AST are enzymes that are manufactured by many cells, including liver cells; when these cells are damaged or destroyed, these enzymes leak into the bloodstream. Thus, they may be present in high concentrations in your blood if you have any number of different liver disorders. Marked elevations usually are seen with acute viral infections of the liver or acute damage to the liver from drugs or toxins.

I've found that many patients and some doctors pay undue attention to ALT and AST levels. This can be a mistake, because with hepatitis C, the actual level of these liver enzymes really doesn't correlate with the severity of the disease (which can be best determined by a liver biopsy). For instance, I might on a given day see two consecutive patients with chronic HCV infection. One may have ALT and AST levels that are two times the upper limit of normal. A subsequent biopsy may confirm moderately advanced disease. The other patient may have ALT and AST levels that are four times the upper limit of normal, but fortunately his or her biopsy may reveal only very mild disease. Moreover, some people with chronic hepatitis C have persistently normal ALT and AST values, and yet their biopsy results indicate fairly advanced disease!

The ALT and AST values also can fluctuate quite a bit without any obvious explanation (the patient is not drinking alcohol, for example). Indeed, before we had the hepatitis C antibody test and we used to call this virus non-A, non-B viral hepatitis, these kinds of cyclical fluctuations were often a clue to doctors that the patient was suffering from non-A, non-B viral hepatitis (now called hepatitis C).

These two enzymes do reflect the level of a person's liver necrosis; that is, the number of cells that are dying and allowing enzymes to leak into the bloodstream. However, sometimes elevations of these two "liver" enzymes are attributable not to liver disease at all but rather to muscle injury. ALT and AST are found in body tissues other than the liver, so damage to these tissues can result in elevated levels of these enzymes in the blood. Each year I see several patients who are sent to me for a second or third opinion with the diagnosis of "unexplained chronic liver disease" (deemed so because of long-lasting elevations in the two liver enzyme levels). I find no evidence of liver disease, and I perform a simple blood test called creatine phosphokinase (CPK, or CK). An elevated CPK level suggests a muscle problem. Indeed, the patient may turn out to have a muscle disorder that is masquerading as a liver disorder. Likewise, a person with bona fide chronic liver disease may injure her muscles from strenuous running or heavy weight lifting. This injury can elevate the AST and ALT levels and fool the physician into thinking that the patient is having a flare-up of her liver problem.

CBC AND PROTHROMBIN TIME. Two other important laboratory tests that your physician will check are called complete blood count (CBC) and prothrombin time (PT). Your CBC is significant because if you have advanced chronic HCV infection, you also may have anemia (a reduced red blood cell count). The other test, PT, measures one important facet of your liver function, which is the production of blood-clotting factors. If your PT is elevated, there are two possibilities: the first is that you have significant liver disease that has altered your blood-clotting mechanism, and the second is that you have an easily correctable vitamin K deficiency. This deficiency can occur for many reasons, including the recent use of antibiotics.

To determine whether you have this more manageable problem, your doctor may give you a few injections of vitamin K and then check your PT again. If it corrects to normal, vitamin K deficiency was responsible for your abnormal test result. If your PT remains elevated, though, or there is only a marginal improvement in the test result, then the prolonged elevation of your PT was caused by liver disease.

SERUM ALBUMIN. I tell my patients to think of the liver as a factory that synthesizes a variety of products, including a protein called albumin. If your albumin is low, you may have liver disease, but several other factors may be responsible as well. For instance, you may be malnourished, or you may have lost excessive albumin from your kidneys because of a condition called nephrotic syndrome.

Albumin also can be lost from a leaky gastrointestinal tract. This problem, which is called protein-losing enteropathy, may be related to a condition known as sprue (or "celiac sprue") or inflammatory bowel disease.

BILIRUBIN. Your doctor also will check your level of bilirubin, a bile pigment found in your blood. If one of the symptoms of your HCV infection is yellow discoloration of your skin and the whites of your eyes (jaundice, or "yellow jaundice"), you will have an increased serum bilirubin value. This is an important test result, because a rising bilirubin level may indicate that your liver disease is getting worse.

ALKALINE PHOSPHATASE. Another blood test that's part of the routine liver function profile measures another enzyme produced in the liver— alkaline phosphatase. The alkaline phosphatase level can go up with several liver disorders, but in general, people with hepatitis C infection do not have significant elevations of this enzyme. If you do have a marked elevation in your alkaline phosphatase level, you may have cholestatic liver disease (blockage of bile flow in the liver). This disease may be accompanied by jaundice and itching.

ALPHA-FETOPROTEIN. If your chronic HCV infection has progressed to cirrhosis, you have an increased chance (approximately 1 to 4 percent per year) of developing primary cancer of the liver (also called primary hepatocellular carcinoma, or hepatoma). Although this possibility may sound frightening, it's important to keep in mind that five to ten years after the diagnosis of chronic HCV infection and cirrhosis, you have an 80 to 90 percent chance of *not* developing liver cancer.

A screening regimen that doctors commonly use to look for liver cancer is a combination of the alpha-fetoprotein (AFP) blood test and an ultrasound of the liver. AFP, a plasma protein, is strikingly elevated in most patients with liver cancer. *Not all elevations in this plasma protein signal the presence of liver cancer, however!* AFP also can be elevated just because the liver is regenerating (healing itself) in response to some type of injury. Elevated or increased AFP levels are also a normal phenomenon during pregnancy. If your AFP level is high, then, your doctor will do some additional tests to find out why.

IRON.   Your doctor also may check the level of iron in your blood (this is called your serum iron) and the amount of iron that your body is storing (this form of iron is called ferritin).

If these levels are elevated, you may have "iron overload." This condition can occur with a variety of liver disorders, including hemochromatosis (see chapter 11); alcoholic liver disease and nonalcoholic steatohepatitis, or NASH (both are described in chapter 8); and porphyria cutanea tarda (see page 210). Indeed, decades ago, at some hospitals, serum iron was used as a "liver function test" to look for liver disease before we had ready access to tests such as ALT and AST.

If you have HCV infection along with mild elevations of iron stores within your liver, you may have a less favorable response to interferon than you would otherwise. If this is the case, you may benefit from a process called de-ironing, or phlebotomy (blood letting). I'll talk about this medieval-sounding, though sometimes helpful, procedure in the next chapter.

RADIOLOGIC TESTS

In addition to a physical examination and blood tests to assess the effects of your HCV infection, your liver specialist may order one or more radiologic tests to take a closer look at your liver.

Ultrasound

Ultrasound is a safe, painless diagnostic procedure that uses very high-frequency sound waves, rather than X rays, to create a picture of the internal structures of the body. If you have chronic HCV infection, your liver specialist may use ultrasound to help him choose an appropriate liver biopsy site; to determine whether or not you have ascites; to explore the cause of your jaundice; or to look for evidence of liver cancer. If your physician orders this test and you're curious about how to prepare for it, turn back to chapter 2 for more details.

BEFORE A LIVER BIOPSY. If your doctor performs a common form of liver biopsy called a needle biopsy, he will likely use percussion to choose the spot from which a very small piece of your liver tissue will be taken; that is, he will tap your upper right side and listen to determine precisely where your lung and liver are situated. Once your doctor has chosen an appropriate biopsy site, he may mark it with a pen and then use an ultrasound probe to confirm that this chosen spot is suitable.

On rare occasions, a person's gallbladder will be seated high up in the liver, or she may have a small, benign tumor of the liver called a hemangioma. When a physician does a liver biopsy, he will want to make sure that the needle isn't directed toward the gallbladder or tumor.

IF YOU MAY HAVE ASCITES. One complication of advanced liver disease is fluid accumulation in the abdomen that can cause you to gain weight and look bloated or "pregnant." In this condition, called ascites, more fluid builds up from the surface of the liver and the intestines than the body's lymphatic system can handle.

If there is any question of whether you have ascites, your doctor will obtain an ultrasound. If ascites is confirmed, your physician then will obtain a sample of the ascitic fluid to try to figure out whether liver scarring (cirrhosis), infection, malignancy, or something else is causing the fluid to accumulate.

IF YOU HAVE JAUNDICE. An ultrasound examination is also an important routine test that can help sort out whether your jaundice is due to a problem within your liver or to obstruction of the bile ducts that come out of your liver and enter your small intestine.

TO SCREEN FOR LIVER CANCER. Finally, as I said earlier, if you have HCV infection and you have developed cirrhosis, you have an increased risk of developing a type of liver cancer called hepatoma. Ultrasound examinations may well make it possible to diagnose this type of tumor at a very early stage, when the chances of successful surgical removal are highest.

Generally, if you have developed cirrhosis due to HCV infection, you should have an ultrasound examination of your liver regularly (approximately every 6 months) to screen for hepatoma. In addition to these ultrasound examinations, an alpha-fetoprotein (AFP) blood test can be done every four months or so to check for this specific tumor marker in your blood. I do these tests in the expectation and hope that no tumor will be found, but if such a mass is found in an early stage, it could be removed surgically.

Computed Tomographic Scanning and Magnetic Resonance Imaging

A computed axial tomographic (CAT) scan uses X rays to view the bones and organs inside your body and to create two- and three-dimensional pictures of them. Liver specialists do not routinely do CAT scans of the liver for people with chronic HCV infection. However, if your doctor sees something suspicious on an ultrasound (such as a blockage or a tumor), he or she may obtain a CAT scan or another test known as magnetic resonance imaging (MRI). MRI is similar to CAT, except that it uses radio waves and a strong magnetic field rather than X rays to generate two- and three-dimensional images of the inner structures of the body.

In rare instances, your physician also may obtain a CAT scan or an MRI of your liver instead of doing a liver biopsy. He may choose to do this because you've had a liver biopsy in the past that resulted in substantial pain, discomfort, or internal bleeding, or if only a small amount of liver tissue was obtained. Please note that these are *rare* complications.

Your doctor may also opt for these radiologic tests over a liver biopsy if you have an underlying bleeding disorder such as hemophilia, a severe bleeding tendency for some other reason, or a lot of free fluid (ascites) within your abdomen.

LIVER BIOPSY

You may wonder why less-invasive tests like CAT and MRI aren't done routinely instead of a liver biopsy to determine what's happening with your liver. The answer is that with few exceptions, these radiologic scans are not good substitutes for a biopsy; the only definitive way to determine whether your liver disease is mild, moderate, or severe is to examine your liver tissue itself under the microscope.

If you're getting ready to undergo a liver biopsy, in chapter 2 you'll find a step-by-step description of what you can expect.

ENDOSCOPY

If your liver biopsy shows that you have severe scarring (cirrhosis), or if your CAT scan suggests features of cirrhosis (such as a distorted, nodular liver, an enlarged spleen, ascites, and prominent veins around your liver and spleen), your liver specialist will recommend that you undergo a test called endoscopy. Endoscopy is done to look for engorged veins called varices in your esophagus. This test is very important, because bleeding from these varices is a potentially life-threatening condition.

Before this procedure, you will be given topical anesthesia and adequate intravenous sedation. A fiberoptic instrument then will be inserted through your mouth into your esophagus and stomach, and the endoscopist will be able to tell from images transmitted to a screen whether or not you have varices. This test has an extremely low complication rate. To find out more about endoscopy and what you can do to prepare for it, see chapter 2.

What if varices are found? Your liver specialist may prescribe a drug called propranolol (Inderal) to decrease your risk of bleeding from these engorged veins (see chapter 9).

Now that you have a better idea of what the symptoms and diagnosis of HCV infection and its complications are like, in the next chapter I'll tell you about treatment options for this liver disease.

6

....

Hepatitis C: Treatment

If you've been diagnosed with hepatitis C, your doctor should be able to tell you whether your disease is mild, moderate, or severe. Your treatment options will be determined by the severity of your disease.

MILD DISEASE

If you have mild disease, there are a couple of options. You can choose to start drug therapy, or you can wait—it's an individual decision. To say that all people with mild HCV infection should be treated would be incorrect, and to state that all people with mild disease should not be treated also would be incorrect. There is no right answer written in bold letters—it's not black and white.

Although this is an important decision and I don't want to make light of it, as Yogi Berra once advised, "If you come to a fork in the road, take it." But should you go left or right? Let's look at your choices.

DRUG THERAPY

The first option is to try the drug therapy that's currently available— combination therapy with the drugs interferon and ribavirin. I endorse this option for most patients if they have a lot of stability in their lives; that is, if they're not overstressed by a demanding job, under pressure to finish a Ph.D. dissertation, or waking up every few hours at night to feed a newborn, and if they're not drinking alcohol and don't have any trouble keeping medical appointments.

Mild HCV infection could be more responsive to treatment than more severe forms of the disease. In fact, if the results of two blood tests show a favorable HCV genetic strain (genotype) and an HCV-RNA viral load that is less than 2 million copies per ml, then the success of treatment with six months of combination therapy can be as high as 70 percent. So it may be worthwhile to give these medications a try. You don't have to commit to a certain number of months of treatment. If you take interferon and ribavirin therapy, but experience significant side effects and inconveniences (see pages 85–89), you can talk with your doctor about stopping treatment and take comfort in the knowledge that eventually better medicines will become available.

GOING WITHOUT TREATMENT

If you're doing well and you truly have mild HCV (as ascertained by liver biopsy), and if there's a lot of stress or strife in your life, then you might decide to defer treatment for six months to a year until you feel up to undergoing treatment and your family is able to provide you with the support that you'll need. If this is the case, your doctors will want to follow your illness carefully. You should alternate your visits to your primary care physician and your hepatologist or gastroenterologist so that you are seeing a doctor every six months.

Your doctors will perform periodic blood tests. You also most likely will need to undergo a liver biopsy approximately two years after your last one. If prior to that two-year point you decide to start treatment with interferon/ribavirin or a better treatment that becomes available, you can begin drug therapy without getting another liver biopsy. Or, if you wait two years and your repeat biopsy shows that your disease has progressed, you can start treatment at that time.

ADVANCED DISEASE

At the other end of the spectrum, if your infection has led to advanced liver scarring (cirrhosis), you may be a candidate for liver transplantation. Hepatitis C is now the number-one reason for this surgical procedure in the United States. In liver transplant centers for adults, approximately one-third of all liver transplants are performed for patients who have chronic hepatitis C with cirrhosis and complications. If your disease is this severe, however, you should be encouraged to know that about 70 percent of people in your situation continue to do very well five years after a liver transplant. Chapter 13 describes this operation in more detail.

This chapter is devoted to the *nonsurgical* treatments that may be recommended for you if you have chronic hepatitis C. These treatments include combination drug therapy with interferon and ribavirin (Rebetron); a drug called amantadine; and a procedure called phlebotomy, or iron reduction therapy. In this chapter I'll also address diet, emotional support, "alternative" remedies, and emerging therapies.

REBETRON

As I said in chapter 3, interferon is a synthetic form of a virus-fighting protein that naturally occurs in our bodies. Interferon works by interfering with the multiplication, or replication, of viruses. Sometimes it can prevent the progression of scarring, or fibrosis, and it may permit the regression of already-existing scar tissue. Until recently, one form of this substance, alpha-interferon (also called interferon A) was the only treatment for HCV infection approved by the U.S. Food and Drug Administration (FDA).

In June 1998 the FDA approved a combination of the drugs interferon and ribavirin for people with chronic HCV infection who initially responded well to interferon treatment, but then relapsed when the treatment was stopped. The success rate of this combined drug therapy, marketed in this country as Rebetron, is a promising 50 percent for such individuals. Most gastroenterologists and hepatologists are now using this combination treatment right off the bat for people who have been newly diagnosed with hepatitis C. That's because for people who have never taken interferon, the success rate of Rebetron can range from 30 to 70 percent (depending primarily upon the patient's genotype). These results stand in stark contrast to the 10 to 20 percent success rate of interferon alone.

PRECAUTIONS

Before you can begin treatment with Rebetron, your doctor will do a complete battery of tests. Any of the following findings could preclude treatment with these drugs:

- Very low blood platelet count (because of a risk of bleeding)
- Very low white blood cell (WBC) count (because of a risk of infection)
- A low hematocrit (because of a risk of anemia)
- Active autoimmune disease (such as rheumatoid arthritis or systemic lupus erythematosus)
- Severe or unremitting depression

Also, if you are or may become pregnant, you must not use Rebetron because animal studies have indicated that this drug can lead to significant birth defects and in some cases even the death of the fetus. Therefore, you must have a negative pregnancy test before you can begin treatment, and if you are a woman of childbearing age, you must use effective contraception during treatment and for six months afterward. If you are a man, you also must use contraception for this length of time because the drug may have an unhealthy effect on sperm. In addition to these warnings, the manufacturer of Rebetron has issued specific warnings for people with renal dysfunction (because this drug is excreted through the kidneys) and cardiovascular disease.

ADMINISTRATION OF REBETRON

If your workup shows no factors that would stand in the way of treatment, you can begin to take these medicines. At the time of this writing, Rebetron, which is manufactured by the Schering-Plough Corporation, is the only FDA-approved interferon/ribavirin combination. It is administered as a combination of interferon A injections and oral ribavirin medication (ribavirin should not be used alone). It comes as a two-week supply, and dosages are determined by body weight.

Prior to starting treatment, you will need to learn to give yourself subcutaneous injections. Turn back to pages 36–37 for some suggestions about how to do this with minimal discomfort. Your physician will monitor your blood tests carefully and frequently while you are taking interferon and ribavirin. The box below provides a schedule of when these various blood tests are generally performed. (For a more detailed discussion of these different types of blood tests, see chapter 2.)

SIDE EFFECTS OF REBETRON THERAPY

About 80 to 90 percent of patients are able to take interferon or interferon/ribavirin with tolerable side effects. In fact, you may be surprised that you can continue working full-time while taking these medications. However, sometimes serious side effects occur; if they do, you should contact your physician immediately. In addition to the potential side

---

Laboratory Tests That Will Be Done during Rebetron Treatment

Week 1, 2, 4, then monthly:
- Complete blood count (CBC)
- Platelet count
- Liver function tests, or LFTs (these include alanine transaminase [ALT] and aspartate transaminase [AST], prothrombin time, albumin, bilirubin, and alkaline phosphatase)

During Week 8:
- CBC
- Platelet count
- LFTs
- Thyroid-stimulating hormone (TSH)

At 12 weeks and at the end of treatment:
- HCV-RNA polymerase chain reaction (PCR) test

Pregnancy tests monthly *in women of childbearing age for the duration of treatment and six months after treatment. If you are taking Rebetron, these pregnancy tests are mandatory.*

effects of interferon therapy (such as a flu-like illness, loss of appetite, irritability, and depression; see pages 37–40), if you're taking ribavirin you may experience symptoms of anemia, itching, nausea and weight loss, coughing, and decreased libido.

Hemolytic Anemia

A condition called hemolytic anemia can occur in people who are taking Rebetron. This condition is related to a decreased number of red blood cells. Because of this potential side effect, your physician will monitor your blood counts one, two, and four weeks after you start treatment, and then monthly.

What does hemolytic anemia feel like? Generally this side effect occurs during the first month of treatment. You may feel fatigued and experience shortness of breath. If you have these symptoms, you should call your doctor.

Approximately 10 percent of people who are taking Rebetron develop *significant* anemia; that is, their hemoglobin level drops to less than 10 g/dl (grams per deciliter); the normal range is 14–18 g/dl for men and 12–16 g/dl for women. This condition is reversible; that is, following discontinuation of Rebetron therapy, blood counts will gradually return to baseline values.

Itching and Rash

Itching also occurs in approximately 10 percent of people who take Rebetron, but it's usually not severe. You might have a rash that's localized to one area, or it may appear all over your body.

Drinking a lot of fluids will keep your skin supple and less prone to irritation. Oatmeal-based soaps and lotions can be very soothing to the skin as well. You also may find that it helps to pat yourself dry with a towel after bathing. If these measures fail, talk to your doctor about topical creams or antihistamines that may help to alleviate this particular side effect.

It's possible that this itching is not related to the Rebetron at all. Or, if the drug is the culprit, it may be exacerbating a previously mild disorder such as eczema or psoriasis. For this reason, referral to a dermatologist may be necessary if one is experiencing a severe or bothersome skin problem.

Nausea and Loss of Appetite

Nausea occurs in up to 50 percent, and a loss of appetite in approximately 20 percent, of people who take Rebetron. These side effects tend to be worse during the first month of treatment. Then, thankfully, they usually dissipate. You can manage these effects by having dry crackers and bread accessible to curb the nausea. Avoid milk products and greasy foods.

These side effects tend to come and go, so that you could feel nauseated in the early morning, but be well and hungry by noon. If this is the case, don't make the mistake of having something greasy like a cheeseburger for lunch, because the nausea may quickly return! Be careful about what you eat until you haven't had this side effect for several days in a row.

If you lose your appetite, try to break your meals into smaller portions and eat throughout the day. For example, eat something every two hours. A half of a sandwich or a nutritious cereal bar are some portable nutritious foods. In addition to minimizing fatigue, light exercise is also a good way to stimulate your appetite.

Cough

Very infrequently, patients develop a cough while undergoing Rebetron treatment. We don't know why this happens. Cough suppressants can help.

Decreased Libido

You may experience a loss of sexual desire while you are taking combination interferon/ribavirin therapy. This could be secondary to other side effects or it may be due to the stress that you are under because of the HCV infection itself.

Communication with your partner is critical. Tell him or her how you are feeling. HCV support groups also can be helpful. If you join one of these groups and bring your loved one, you probably will feel less isolated and perhaps closer to your partner as well.

DISCONTINUATION OF THERAPY

Your doctor will pay close attention to any side effects that you might be having from this treatment. You can help her in this process by informing her of all side effects that you are aware of. If you experience severe depression or psychiatric problems (again, these side effects are rare) or other intolerable side effects, your physician may discontinue your treatment with interferon/ribavirin. She also *may* stop your treatment with this type of therapy if:

- Your white blood count (WBC) falls below 1200
- Your neutrophil count falls below 500 (neutrophils are a type of white blood cell)
- Your platelet count falls below 30,000
- Your hemoglobin (Hgb) level is less than 8.5 g/dl

Again, experts don't always agree totally about factors that should preclude or cause discontinuation of treatment, so you should talk with your doctor about his or her recommendations.

RESPONSES TO REBETRON

Physicians measure the success of combination interferon and ribavirin therapy according to a person's specific biochemical, virologic, and histologic responses to these drugs. A positive *biochemical response* means that when your blood is tested, your plasma ALT value will have normalized from its previously elevated level. Remember that liver enzymes like ALT leak into the bloodstream from damaged liver cells. So a decreased level of ALT in your blood will mean that the virus is doing less or no damage to your liver. A positive *virologic response* means that when you have an HCV-RNA-PCR test (see pages 72–73), your physician will not be able to detect any copies of the hepatitis C virus circulating in your bloodstream. Finally, a favorable *histologic response* means that when viewed under a microscope, your liver tissue (from a liver biopsy) will show less inflammation, fewer dead and dying cells (necrosis), and possibly even less scar tissue (fibrosis) than the pretreatment biopsy specimen did.

OUTCOMES OF INTERFERON AND RIBAVIRIN TREATMENT

While you are undergoing treatment, your physician will monitor you regularly with blood tests to see what happens to your viral load (your HCV-RNA level) as well as your ALT level. At the time of this writing, many authorities in the field recommend repeating the HCV-RNA quantitative test three and six months after treatment has been started and checking the ALT level monthly. These repeat tests will show one of the four following outcomes:

- Nonresponse or partial response
- Breakthrough
- Complete but non-sustained response
- Complete and sustained response

This is what it means to have one of these potential outcomes:

Nonresponse or Partial Response

If your gastroenterologist or hepatologist says that you have a "nonresponse" or "partial response" to Rebetron therapy, she may mean that:

- Your ALT level has not become normal (so presumably the virus is still present and causing liver damage); or
- Your RNA test remains positive (i.e., HCV is still present in your bloodstream).

If this is your body's response to these medicines, your treatment strategy will have to be altered and you may need to consider other therapies, such as a different kind or higher dose of interferon or other new medications that are for the most part only available in clinical trials. If you fall into this group of "nonresponders" or "partial responders," though, there is some encouraging news about the potential benefits from the interferon that was administered. A number of studies have shown that although some people may not appear to benefit from interferon treatment with a favorable biochemical and virologic response (that is, the ALT level did not normalize, and there continues to be a detectable level of virus in the blood on the RNA test), the liver cells actually look healthier histologically (that is, when examined under the microscope).

In fact, a liver biopsy may show that the rate of scar tissue (fibrosis) progression has slowed down. It's thus possible that interferon is having a helpful effect in people whom we traditionally have classified as "nonresponders." Perhaps we need to change our definition of nonresponse! A few studies also indicate that for people with advanced disease (cirrhosis), interferon may decrease the risk of developing liver cancer. This may be how: angiogenesis, a unique mechanism that allows new blood vessels to form from existing ones, enables cancerous tumors to grow. Interferon may disrupt this mechanism, and in doing so may protect people from developing such tumors. Dr. Judah Folkman at Children's Hospital in Boston has been studying angiogenesis in a variety of disorders for several decades and has contributed remarkably to our understanding of this phenomenon.

These exciting advances hold great promise for patients with advanced liver disease due to hepatitis C. In the near future, it is likely that large-scale, well-designed clinical trials will examine whether low-dose maintenance interferon for such patients does indeed prevent liver cancer.

Breakthrough

The second possible outcome of Rebetron treatment, a "breakthrough," is the most disappointing. A breakthrough means that during the early part of treatment, your ALT level normalizes, but as the treatment continues, things change course, and your ALT becomes elevated again. The mechanism of this change is not clear. You may have developed antibodies to interferon, or the virus may have mutated. Fortunately, this outcome is rare: less than 5 percent of people will experience breakthrough disease.

Complete but Nonsustained Response

If you have a "complete but nonsustained response" to Rebetron, your ALT levels will decrease to a normal range, and your HCV-RNA-PCR tests will be negative (i.e., the virus will not be detected in your blood) during treatment. However, this response is temporary, and when you stop taking these medicines, you will soon relapse (in other words, your liver enzyme levels will become abnormal again and your HCV-RNA-PCR test will become positive).

The relapse may manifest as early as a few weeks after you have stopped the initial course of treatment. On rare occasions, the relapse occurs many months later.

Complete and Sustained Response

With the best, "complete and sustained response" to treatment, the ALT level in your blood will be normal, and your HCV-RNA-PCR test will be negative six months after you have stopped treatment. You will not have a relapse of your infection several years out. A number of my patients who successfully completed treatment with interferon many years ago now have completely normal ALT levels and negative PCR tests.

I've found that such "responders" to treatment also appear to have a significant improvement in their quality of life, not only because their symptoms have improved but because worries about their health, fears about infecting others, work-related concerns, and uncertainty about the future also abate when this favorable outcome is achieved.

My patients often ask if we actually can get rid of this virus or if we can suppress it completely. Although in the past we've been hesitant to use the word *cure* for hepatitis C, we now have extremely encouraging results: one study from Clichy, France, followed eighty patients with a sustained response to interferon treatment for approximately one to eight years. Approximately 95 percent of these people had normal serum ALT levels, and no detectable virus in their blood. Twenty-seven of these patients also underwent repeat liver biopsies one to five years after stopping interferon treatment. In all twenty-seven, there was no detectable trace of the virus in the liver tissue.

Dr. Jay Hoofnagle, a senior and eminent investigator at the U.S. National Institutes of Health, and colleagues reported on a very important study. They followed ten patients who had been taking alpha-interferon therapy from 1984 through 1986. Five out of ten of these patients, like the patients in the Clichy study, were "sustained responders." Now, twelve to fourteen years later, these five patients have no symptoms of HCV infection; they have normal liver enzyme levels, they have negative RNA-PCR markers for the virus, and their repeat liver biopsies show no significant scar tissue. These results in responders with interferon monotherapy (that is, the drug was used alone, not in combination with ribavirin) are indeed remarkably gratifying!

WHAT IF YOU RELAPSE?

What if, after stopping Rebetron, you have a relapse—that is, your PCR level becomes positive again? You should see your liver specialist, who will decide with you whether to forego treatment for now and await better therapies that may come along; to enroll in a clinical trial to try a new drug for HCV that is under development; or to take low-dose maintenance interferon on a long-term basis (as long as it is tolerated). With the latter option, although the virus may not be eradicated, there may be suppression of the virus and a significant decrease in disease activity.

PHLEBOTOMY

Phlebotomy, also called iron reduction therapy or bloodletting, is another treatment option that you may hear about if you have hepatitis C.

Your liver stores most of the iron found in your body, but sometimes excessive amounts of this trace metal can build up in your liver tissue and create a condition known as iron overload. This buildup can be harmful and can affect the way in which your body responds to drugs like interferon. Therefore, your doctor may recommend that you have a certain amount of blood drawn on a regular basis in order to reduce your iron level and keep it in a normal range. This technique, which is used primarily for people with a liver condition called hemochromatosis, is described in more detail in chapter 11.

If you appear to have a "near complete response" to interferon—that is, your ALT level falls but does not completely normalize, and your viral load drops dramatically from, for example, 3 million to 8,000 copies of the virus—and if you have any suggestion of iron overload on blood tests or a liver biopsy, phlebotomy may be an important adjunct to drug therapy. I also have seen a few patients in whom phlebotomy treatment involving the removal of a total of 6 to 8 units of blood has led to both normalization of the patient's plasma ALT level and elimination of the virus on RNA-PCR. In rare instances, this has happened without interferon or combination interferon-ribavirin therapy! A better understanding of the beneficial role of iron reduction therapy is clearly needed.

Finally, if your doctor has found that you have too much iron in your body, you certainly should not take iron supplements. I also would advise you to limit your consumption of foods that are high in iron (such as red meat and iron-fortified cereals).

AMANTADINE

An initial pilot study showed some promise for treatment of HCV infection with an antiviral drug called amantadine. It appears to be a well-tolerated medication; that is, there are few side effects. However, my limited experience with amantadine and the experiences of a number of my colleagues throughout the country, each of whom have prescribed amantadine for some of their patients, have been somewhat disappointing. Well-designed large-scale studies need to be done to ascertain whether this drug by itself or in combination with other drugs has any potential benefit.

DIET

There is no proven "diet cure" for hepatitis C. I can offer you some recommendations, though. Undoubtedly the most important advice is that you should avoid alcohol completely to prevent further damage to your liver, and you should eat a well-balanced diet. Also, as I just mentioned, if your iron level is too high, you should limit your consumption of iron-rich foods.

The answer to the question of how much protein you should eat is less straightforward. Protein is essential for regeneration of liver cells in people who do not have cirrhosis. However, if your HCV infection has led to cirrhosis and you are at risk for a complication known as hepatic encephalopathy (see chapter 9), you may need to restrict the amount of animal protein (meat, fish, eggs, and dairy products) in your diet. Your doctor should be able to advise you about the amount of protein that you should consume.

You also should ask your doctor for advice about a weight-reducing diet (and exercise) if you have HCV infection and you are overweight, because it's possible that obesity is causing some damage to your liver. Features of this type of damage may be evident on a liver biopsy.

Lastly, I recommend that my patients take 800 international units of vitamin E daily because it may retard scarring (fibrosis) within the liver.

EMOTIONAL SUPPORT

Although the support of your family and friends won't cure your hepatitis C infection, having a trusted companion with you when you're discussing your diagnosis and treatment with your doctor and sharing the ups and downs of this long-term illness with your family members certainly can be of tremendous help.

Your emotional health also can be bolstered by participating in an HCV support group sponsored by your local hospital. The American Liver Foundation and other such organizations may be able to provide you with invaluable help and information, too. Lastly, you may be surprised to know that a few pharmaceutical companies have programs for people with HCV. Some even offer free medications if you fulfill certain eligibility requirements. If you're interested in finding out more about these programs, you may wish to start with the list of resources at the back of this book.

ALTERNATIVE TREATMENTS

Although "alternative" medicine is sometimes called "nontraditional" medicine, it actually encompasses a wide range of healing traditions from all over the world. Some of these traditions include:

- *Indian Ayurvedic medicine,* which embraces yoga, herbs, and fasting
- *Chinese medicine,* which may incorporate acupuncture, massage, herbs, and treatments to keep yin and yang energy in balance in the body
- *Naturopathy,* which promotes massage, diet, and the use of natural forces such as water, heat, and light instead of medicines
- *Homeopathy,* which involves the use of small amounts of drugs that, if given to a healthy person, may create symptoms of the disease being treated

A growing number of Americans are visiting specialists who advocate these alternative healing methods, and a recent article in the *Journal of the American Medical Association* indicated that 15 million Americans take both herbal medications and traditional prescription medications at the same time.

You may be curious about whether any of these herbal remedies might cure your hepatitis C infection. You may even be trying some of them instead of (or in addition to) interferon or Rebetron treatment. I'd like to share with you both my interest in and concern about the use of alternative therapies.

DO ALTERNATIVE TREATMENTS WORK?

Many of my patients ask, "Can these remedies help?" I tell them that some of them *may* help. The scientific community, which previously was most skeptical of alternative treatments, is now at least open to the possibility that some of these measures may have beneficial effects. There are divisions of alternative medicine at some of the most prestigious medical schools in the world. Undoubtedly, in the near future, research looking at these alternative methods will answer the question of whether these therapies have benefit.

For example, very recently in *Hepatology*, the official journal of the American Association for the Study of Liver Diseases, some investigators described their research involving Sho-saiko-to (also known as Xiano-Chai-Hu-Tang), an herbal medicine that has been used in China for thousands of years for chronic hepatitis. In this study, rats were given a compound that causes the development of liver scarring (hepatic fibrosis). In rats who also were given Sho-saiko-to, there was very powerful suppression of hepatic fibrosis. This is an exciting study that eventually *might* have some potential for humans. More research needs to be done to determine the actual utility and safety of this compound.

An accompanying editorial in the same issue of *Hepatology* was entitled "Sho-saiko-to: The Right Blend of Traditional Oriental Medicine and Liver Cell Biology." In it, two Belgian professors acclaim the study of this herbal agent. They note, "Broadening our horizons by critically exploring age-old remedies may still yield important information. We should not overlook these opportunities in our zeal to embrace technology-driven drug discovery."

I agree that scientists should be exploring these herbal medicines. If such remedies turn out to be of even partial benefit, and if they are safe and inexpensive, they could provide a substantial boost to the psychological well-being of the individual. Even agents that may decrease the level of a person's liver enzymes (but do not eradicate the virus from the body) may contribute in a meaningful fashion to his or her psychological welfare.

I personally practice meditation twice a day, and I'm very receptive to the potential of alternative or complementary medicines. Nevertheless, every time I hear about somebody who has responded to alternative remedies, there is a bit of a tug. On the one hand, I'm intrigued by the possibility that this agent might work. On the other hand, my scientific skepticism reminds me that before we embrace some of these alternative regimens, we need to do large-scale studies. We need to apply the same yardsticks to natural remedies that we do to traditional drugs.

Not long ago, I had this sort of mixed reaction when I read that the country musician Naomi Judd, who may have contracted hepatitis C while working as a nurse more than ten years ago, has had some success with a compound called thymus extract. In her autobiography,

Love Can Build a Bridge, she says that since her diagnosis, she has pursued various methods to help her body fight HCV. She has tried to improve her diet by eating yogurt and organic produce and she has taken extra vitamins (A, B, C, and E) and minerals (zinc, selenium, folic acid, magnesium, and potassium), as well as extra beta-carotene and other antioxidants. She also has tried guided imagery, progressive muscle relaxation, meditation, and acupuncture. In addition to these dietary and stress-reducing practices, she has taken herbal supplements such as thymus extract, and she says that these supplements have dramatically improved her health.

I too believe that good nutrition is important for all patients, and that visual imagery, massage, and acupuncture may have some benefit—and I'm personally delighted that Naomi Judd has found thymus extract to be helpful. Yet because she also has taken interferon, it's impossible to say whether the alternative remedies that she has tried have been responsible for any beneficial changes in her condition. Secondly, even if she had *not* taken interferon and a sensitive HCV-RNA-PCR test showed that the virus was no longer present in her blood, we still wouldn't say that thymus extract is a cure for all patients with HCV, because what we're looking at is just one person's experience with this remedy.

"Traditional," FDA-approved drugs are deemed acceptable for public use only after they have been tested and found to work in scores of patients, not just in one or even a few individuals. Although some studies have been done to explore the potential effectiveness of remedies like thymus extract (see pages 102–103), no large-scale clinical trials have proven that thymus extract can benefit many patients.

Now I'd like to share with you some of the other thoughts that I have about herbal remedies.

They're Not Scientifically Validated

The use of herbal remedies concerns me not just because their effectiveness has not been proven for many people, but because in some cases these agents have hardly been scientifically tested at all. In a recent publication called *Self Healing,* the feature article was devoted to "natural help for hepatitis." In it, Andrew Weil, a respected guru of alternative medicine and author of *Spontaneous Healing* and *Eight Weeks to Optimum Health,* recounted the story of a friend of his named Susan who was diagnosed as having chronic hepatitis C. She had seen a few specialists who had recommended taking interferon, but she didn't want to take this drug because of its "major flu-like side effects and a response rate of only 20 to 30 percent."

Dr. Weil advised Susan to make some specific nutritional and lifestyle changes. He also referred her to a practitioner of Chinese medicine, who gave her a mixture of Chinese herbs. Three months later, her liver enzyme levels were tested, and they were normal for the first time in twelve years. Six months after that, these enzyme levels remained normal, and she said that she plans to adhere to her herbal treatment program for the foreseeable future.

Although this story indicated that Susan's liver enzyme tests normalized while she was taking Chinese herbal medication, it didn't say what happened to her HCV-RNA levels (that is, how much virus was actually present in her system) or to the health of her liver tissue under the microscope (her "liver histology"). Scientific research into the treatment of HCV infection is rapidly evolving, and the drugs that we already have show great promise. We shouldn't necessarily embrace an alternative remedy that may simply normalize liver enzyme levels when we don't really know what is happening to the person's viral load or liver histology.

Herbal medications may turn out to be beneficial in the treatment of chronic hepatitis C, either on their own or as adjuncts to traditional medicines like interferon and ribavirin. I sincerely hope they do. And I'm pleased that practitioners such as Dr. Weil are talking about complementary therapies for viral hepatitis and bringing about a greater awareness of this epidemic in our country. Perhaps in part because of this heightened attention to such alternative possibilities, scientists will step up their research into the safety and efficacy of these remedies.

REGULATION OF ALTERNATIVE TREATMENTS, AND THEIR POTENTIAL DANGERS

In addition to the fact that they haven't been scientifically validated, another concern that I have with alternative medicines is that they generally don't undergo good quality control or regulation. The active ingredient thus may vary considerably from one preparation to another, and there's no guarantee that these herbal remedies are free of pesticides or other toxins. The lack of scientific scrutiny and regulation of herbal remedies means that even though they may be called "natural" or "herbal," they may not be safe. On occasion patients have developed fatal liver diseases as a consequence of using such treatments.

A number of drugs with ostensible nutritional, medicinal, hypnotic, weight loss, or health aid benefits have been shown to produce significant liver injury. Some can lead to a dangerous form of fatty infiltration of the liver, some to blockage of the veins inside the liver (this is called veno-occlusive disease), and some even to chronic hepatitis and cirrhosis. The herbal products that have been known to cause such problems include comfrey; maté tea; gordolobo herbal tea; Chinese herb preparations such as jin bu huan; germander; chaparral leaf; and margosa oil.

THEY'RE NOT INEXPENSIVE

Finally, in addition to their lack of proven effectiveness and their potential dangers, alternative agents may turn out to be costly (the average price for a month's supply of milk thistle, for example, is about $25). One patient of mine was racking up a monthly bill of close to $300 taking a bunch of herbal drugs and vitamins. She felt empowered, but there was no benefit (her viral load did not decrease), and in reality what she was taking was a pretty hefty "wallet biopsy."

In light of all of these concerns about herbal preparations, what should you do if you're already taking this type of remedy for your HCV infection? You definitely should let your doctor know, because sometimes dangerous drug interactions do occur. It is possible that taking an alternative medicine such as milk thistle may provide some psychological benefit; in that sense, it has some utility. Your gastroenterologist or hepatologist, who best knows your situation, will be able to guide you.

RESEARCH AND HOPE FOR THE FUTURE

PREVENTION

There are currently no vaccines available to prevent hepatitis C infection. However, the CDC Advisory Committee on Immunization Practices recommends that all people with chronic liver disease (including hepatitis C) receive the hepatitis A and B vaccines. That's because hepatitis A or B infection superimposed on chronic hepatitis C can be a very serious disorder and occasionally can lead to a fatal outcome. I do not routinely vaccinate my patients who have HCV, because a lot of them have had previous exposure to and immunity against hepatitis A and B viral infections. Their immunity can be determined by a simple, inexpensive blood test. If a person does not have immunity to these viruses, I recommend that they be given the appropriate vaccine.

Researchers are working on a vaccine for the hepatitis C virus, but it's not yet ready for human trials as of this writing. Initial studies with the vaccine have been disappointing. In the laboratory, chimps inoculated with a particular strain of HCV came down with acute HCV infection and then recovered. Then, in the "rechallenge" phase of the experiment, the chimps became infected again with the same strain of the virus. Although these sobering results bode poorly for the development of an effective vaccine for humans in the near future, progress is being made in this endeavor.

Indeed, recent preliminary reports suggest that scientists in the laboratory have established cell lines that can be transfected with HCV. That means that they can "infect" cells with HCV and then explore the way in which the virus duplicates itself and multiplies. This development should enable researchers to study not only the life cycle of HCV but the mechanism of liver injury as well, and could facilitate the development of effective vaccines.

PROSPECTS FOR FUTURE TREATMENT

Funding and Public Awareness

As Dr. Jerome Groopman noted in a 1998 *New Yorker* article entitled "The Shadow Epidemic," the National Institutes of Health (NIH) spent a total of $1.5 billion, or $1,600 per infected person, in the United States for AIDS research in 1997, but only $25 million, or $6 per infected person, on HCV research. AIDS deaths in the United States have declined dramatically from 43,000 in 1995 to 16,000 in 1997. For us to see similar progress with HCV, clearly funding levels need to increase as the numbers of people who are diagnosed with HCV infection continue to rise.

The president of the American Liver Foundation also has called on the U.S. government to spend more on educating the public and primary care physicians about this disease; to subsidize HCV testing for those at greatest risk of becoming infected; and to establish an HCV information, referral, and support network.

Refinements to Interferon Therapy

Currently two refinements to interferon administration are under clinical investigation. The first, induction therapy, involves administration of daily and sometimes larger than usual doses of interferon (e.g., 5 million units daily rather than 3 million units daily) at the start of treatment for four to eight weeks. Hypothetically, this regimen should be advantageous because HCV multiplies very rapidly, and so it makes sense to try to "knock it out" in the first month or two of treatment.

The second refinement is a product called polyethylene glycol (PEG) interferon, which is given to the patient once a week. This option sounds attractive, too, because it may be better tolerated (since it is given only once a week), and it may be more effective because a steady level of interferon is released slowly from this formulation. One study that was presented at the 1999 annual meeting of the American Association for the Study of Liver Diseases (AASLD) indicated a 30 percent sustained-response success rate when PEG interferon was administered to patients with chronic HCV infection and advanced liver disease (cirrhosis). At the 2000 annual meeting of the AASLD, investigators reported the success rate of combination PEG interferon and ribavirin therapy for 48 weeks to be 40 to 50 percent (sustained response) in patients with genotype 1. Moreover, they reported a 90 percent success rate in patients with genotype 2 or 3.

New Drug Therapies

PROTEASE INHIBITORS. The drugs that appear to be the most promising for the treatment of HCV are the protease inhibitors. Agents like protease, helicase, and polymerase inhibitors interfere with the enzymes necessary for replication of viruses. Protease inhibitors have been used with dramatic success against the AIDS virus; however, the protease inhibitors being used to fight HIV will not work for treating HCV infection. Many scientists worldwide are actively engaged in developing similar but different compounds for HCV, which may become effective against this virus in the next few years.

INTERLEUKIN-10. In a recent pilot study, a new compound called interleukin-10 (IL-10) was found to normalize liver enzymes, decrease the amount of liver inflammation, and reduce the amount of scar tissue (fibrosis) in patients with HCV infection, even though it did not eradicate the virus or produce significant inhibition of viral replication. If large-scale studies bear out these findings, IL-10 would be a most valuable agent in our fight against HCV.

MILK THISTLE. For centuries silymarin, a substance derived from the milk thistle plant, has been used to treat liver diseases. Some studies suggest that it has antioxidant properties. However, a few of my patients who were not suitable candidates for interferon treatment because of significant preexisting depression tried milk thistle as an alternative treatment, and their viral load did not change. Thus, it's possible that this treatment may actually have a detrimental effect. Well-designed scientific studies are needed to see whether milk thistle has any potential benefit for treating HCV infection.

THYMOSIN AND OTHER COMPOUNDS. Researchers are studying a number of compounds, including thymosin, an extract of the thymus gland, for treatment of hepatitis C infection. Results of these studies have been mixed, and further research with large clinical trials is needed. Many of these compounds have been shown to decrease or even normalize the plasma ALT value or decrease viral levels. However, at present, there is no conclusive proof that these agents eradicate the virus, improve liver histology, or favorably alter the natural history of the disease.

SOME FINAL RECOMMENDATIONS

You've been diagnosed with hepatitis C. Perhaps you've already seen a gastroenterologist or hepatologist or have started taking therapy. Let's review some of the most important points that you'll need to keep in mind in the days ahead:

- Be well informed about your disease. Assess all new information, whether it comes from a traditional or alternative medical practitioner, a friend, a colleague, a magazine, or a posting on the Internet, with careful and knowledgeable objectivity. Do not embrace alternative or even new conventional treatments blindly.
- Know what stage of the disease you have. Do you have a mild infection, or is your case of hepatitis C complicated by cirrhosis?
- Garner the support of your family and friends; look into a support group.
- Contact the American Liver Foundation, pharmaceutical companies, and other resources for information and assistance.
- Don't donate blood, organs, tissue, or semen.
- Don't share toothbrushes, razor blades, or nail clippers.
- Practice safe sex.
- Avoid alcohol completely.
- Be sure that, if necessary, you have been vaccinated against hepatitis A and B.
- Notify any dentists, doctors, or other health care workers who may come into contact with your blood that you have HCV infection.
- Take 800 international units of vitamin E daily.
- Insist on seeing a specialist.

SUMMARY

Not too long ago, we called a virus that was neither hepatitis A nor hepatitis B *non-A, non-B hepatitis*. Now we have a name for it: hepatitis C. If you have this virus, your doctor has access to definitive tests that can measure the amount of virus in your body and determine which genetic strain, or genotype, of the virus is affecting you.

Now we have two FDA-approved drugs—interferon and ribavirin—and we have refined the amount and duration of treatment so that when these two drugs are given in combination for six months to a year, the success rate ranges from 33 to 41 percent. Even more encouraging, when this combination is given for six months to patients who have a low viral load and are infected with genotypes 2 or 3, the success rate can be as high as 70 percent. With combination PEG interferon and ribavirin therapy likely to be available in the near future, the success rate approaches 90 percent.

We've made a lot of progress in a very short period of time. Undoubtedly, with all of the attention that the HCV epidemic is receiving in our country and throughout the world, dedicated investigators will make even more important strides in the near future.

7

. . . .

Autoimmune Hepatitis

Last spring, Janet, a forty-eight-year-old teacher, went on vacation to Mexico with her husband, Bill, who is an orthopedic surgeon. A few weeks after they returned to their home in New Hampshire, she began to experience some mild abdominal discomfort and appetite loss. She also felt achy and fatigued, almost as if she had the flu. When Bill noticed that Janet's skin and the whites of her eyes had a yellowish cast, he became concerned that while they were on vacation she might have acquired a viral infection affecting the liver and urged her to see her primary care physician as soon as possible. The next morning, she went to see Dr. Christine Murphy, who noticed Janet's yellowish skin and eyes right away. She examined Janet and found that her liver was enlarged and tender.

Dr. Murphy's clinical impression of jaundice was confirmed by a laboratory blood test that showed a modestly elevated level of bilirubin, the bile pigment that, when present in the blood at an abnormally high level, results in "yellow jaundice." Moreover, the levels of two liver enzymes called alanine transaminase (ALT) and aspartate transaminase (AST) were markedly elevated; these enzyme levels tend to soar with various types of liver disorders, including viral infections and liver damage caused by a number of drugs. However, Janet's prothrombin time, a measure of her blood's clotting abilities and a very important liver function test, was reassuringly normal.

As Dr. Murphy talked with Janet about her medical history, she learned that Janet and Bill had not taken gamma globulin before their trip, even though it protects against the hepatitis A virus (HAV) and is recommended for travelers to areas such as Mexico, where HAV is endemic. Janet also mentioned that Bill was worried that she might have acquired a hepatitis infection. She said that he was regretting that he'd not yet been vaccinated against the hepatitis B virus (HBV), even though it's prudent for all physicians to do so.

As they talked, Dr. Murphy continued to go through a mental checklist of risk factors for viral hepatitis infections. When she asked Janet if she ever ate uncooked seafood (a risk factor for HAV infection), Janet said that recently she'd been on a "sushi kick," and that she and Bill had been going to Japanese restaurants frequently. Given all of these clues—Janet's visit to an area where HAV infection is prevalent and her risk of contracting this virus from eating raw seafood, as well as her husband's potential exposure to HBV in the workplace, and her risk of contracting it from him—Dr. Murphy surmised that her patient probably had an acute infection with either the hepatitis A or B virus. However, when she performed the specific blood tests to look for these viruses, they turned out to be negative. Puzzled, she referred Janet to me for consultation.

When I met Janet, she told me that she had always been fairly healthy, and that she didn't take any medicines regularly. When I asked her about other potential risk factors for certain types of viral hepatitis besides the ones that Dr. Murphy had asked her about, she said that she'd never used intravenous drugs or cocaine, had acupuncture, or gotten a tattoo.

When I examined her, I found that Janet looked tired, but she had no features of chronic liver disease (such as red palms and spiderlike veins on her skin). She was mildly jaundiced, though, and her liver was swollen. She said that it hurt when I palpated the lower edge of her liver, below the right rib cage. I performed some additional blood tests that revealed that Janet's liver enzyme (ALT and AST) levels had risen dramatically and were now at a level that was 50 to 100 times the upper limit of normal! Nevertheless, her prothrombin time (the measure of her blood's clotting ability) remained normal, and fortunately she had no features of liver failure such as hepatic encephalopathy, a condition that can occur when liver function is altered substantially and the liver cannot clear the body of certain toxins such as ammonia. When these toxins accumulate, they can affect the brain and lead to confusion that ranges from mild and subtle changes in mental faculties to frank coma.

Next I ordered two additional blood tests: an antinuclear antibody (ANA) test and an immunoglobulin G (IgG) level. The first was positive, and the second was markedly elevated. When these results were available, I made the diagnosis of a type of liver inflammation (hepatitis) called autoimmune hepatitis and recommended that Janet undergo a liver biopsy to confirm the diagnosis and to find out how extensive her disease was. The liver biopsy revealed that Janet indeed had fairly severe acute hepatitis. When I looked at the biopsy specimen under the microscope, I also saw an increased number of plasma cells—a characteristic sign of autoimmune hepatitis. Fortunately, though, there was no scar tissue (fibrosis).

On the basis of the ANA and IgG blood tests, as well as the liver biopsy results, I concluded with certainty that Janet had autoimmune hepatitis of moderate severity, but that she did not have cirrhosis.

WHAT IS AUTOIMMUNE HEPATITIS?

When I first told Janet about her diagnosis, she was relieved that we had found out what was making her feel unwell, but she had many questions: First of all, she wanted to know what had caused her hepatitis. I told her that autoimmune hepatitis, a rare disease that is seen worldwide, involves a loss of tolerance to one's own liver cells. The body's immune system mounts an attack against these cells, and liver damage ensues.

Janet's eyes widened. "Oh, my cousin had an autoimmune problem—lupus," Janet said. "Are these two diseases related?"

"There's no connection," I assured her, "and don't worry—neither disease is contagious."

Occasionally, viruses (such as hepatitis A) and drugs may trigger autoimmune hepatitis, and it's likely that some people may have a genetic predisposition to this disease. Autoimmune hepatitis accounts for an estimated 5 percent of cases of chronic (or long-term) hepatitis.

Other more common causes of chronic liver inflammation are the hepatitis B and C viruses. Also, rarely, long-term use of certain drugs can lead to chronic hepatitis. These drugs include Aldomet (methyldopa) for high blood pressure; isoniazid (INH) for tuberculosis; and nitrofurantoin, an antibacterial agent often used in the treatment of urinary tract infections. Likewise, chronic hepatitis can be caused by inherited metabolic disorders such as Wilson's disease, in which there is abnormal metabolism of copper in the body (see page 158).

Autoimmune hepatitis was first described by Dr. Waldenstrom in the early 1950s, and it's been known by many names over the years. These include chronic active hepatitis, chronic aggressive hepatitis, juvenile cirrhosis, autoimmune liver disease, plasma cell hepatitis, and lupoid hepatitis (although autoimmune hepatitis is not related to lupus, an inflammatory disorder that affects the body's connective tissue). *Autoimmune hepatitis* is currently the most widely used term for this condition.

This type of hepatitis is not very common; there are only an estimated 100 cases per 1 million Caucasians in North America (unfortunately, accurate figures for other populations are not available). The prevalence is similar to that of systemic lupus erythematosus, or SLE (again, there is no connection between these two conditions) and primary biliary cirrhosis (PBC).

In many ways, Janet was a fairly typical autoimmune hepatitis patient. Ninety percent of people with this disease are female, and it's found most commonly in individuals who are ten to sixty years old.

SYMPTOMS

If you have autoimmune hepatitis, you may have no symptoms, and your doctor may discover this condition in the process of doing routine bloodwork as part of a comprehensive health examination. Or, like Janet, you may have a case of acute hepatitis, or severe inflammation of the liver. You may experience fatigue, malaise, low energy, "depression," loss of appetite, or abdominal discomfort, or you may pass dark urine. Autoimmune hepatitis predominantly affects the liver, but if you have this condition your joints may be painful.

Some patients also develop thyroid abnormalities (most often an underactive thyroid gland, or hypothyroidism) or dry gland syndrome (sicca, or Sjögren's syndrome), which causes dryness in the eyes and mouth. Rarely, inflammatory bowel disease (either ulcerative colitis or Crohn's disease) may be present. If you are a woman, your menstrual periods may stop.

With very severe disease, you may first come to clinical attention because you have something called acute fulminant hepatitis, a serious form of liver failure that comes on like a bolt of lightning and causes mild to severe mental confusion (hepatic encephalopathy) because the liver has stopped purging toxins such as ammonia from the blood.

Finally, your doctor may find that autoimmune hepatitis is the cause of your already well-established case of cirrhosis (liver scarring) and its complications, such as fluid in the abdomen (ascites) or bleeding from prominent veins called varices in your esophagus. In fact, approximately one-half of all patients with severe autoimmune hepatitis who undergo liver biopsies (patients with very mild disease may not have this procedure done) are found to have cirrhosis.

DIAGNOSIS

LABORATORY TESTS

The diagnosis of autoimmune hepatitis requires the performance of simple blood tests such as a complete blood count (CBC), blood-clotting parameters (such as prothrombin time and platelet count), and liver function tests. The latter tests include the liver enzymes alanine transaminase (ALT) and aspartate transaminase (AST), bilirubin, and albumin. These tests are described in more detail in chapter 2. In addition, special blood tests such as those that were performed for Janet should be done; these include the antinuclear antibody (ANA) and serum immunoglobulin (IgG) level.

Hepatitis serologies are performed, too. These blood tests are taken to exclude the hepatitis viruses (A, B, and C) and other illnesses such as Wilson's disease as factors that may be causing your liver inflammation. If these tests show that you are not infected with these viruses and you are not immune to them, you may need to be vaccinated against HAV and HBV, because these infections superimposed on your autoimmune hepatitis could make you very ill. (Unfortunately, at present there is no vaccine available for the hepatitis C virus.)

LIVER BIOPSY

If you are diagnosed with autoimmune hepatitis, your primary care physician may refer you to a specialist in disorders of the gastrointestinal system (a gastroenterologist) or a liver specialist (a hepatologist). Such a specialist may perform a liver biopsy to confirm the diagnosis, stage the extent of your liver injury (the most important thing is to see if cirrhosis is present or absent), and exclude other causes of liver dysfunction. This procedure, which is described in detail in chapter 2, is usually done on an outpatient basis for people with mild liver disease. If your disease is severe, however, you may be admitted to the hospital both for a liver biopsy and to start treatment.

HOW SEVERE IS YOUR AUTOIMMUNE HEPATITIS?

Like every other condition in medicine, autoimmune hepatitis may range from mild to severe disease. The severity is based on a number of factors, including your symptoms, the degree of abnormality of your liver function test results (particularly the level of the liver enzymes ALT and AST, the height of gamma globulin elevation, and the pro-thrombin time), and whether cirrhosis or features of hepatic encepha-lopathy are present.

If you have a mild case of autoimmune hepatitis, you may have only mild elevations of your AST and ALT, a mild elevation in gamma globu-lin, and a positive ANA test. If your liver biopsy also indicates mild dis-ease, you could go without treatment as long as you are monitored closely with regular checkups. Sometimes, even for mild autoimmune hepatitis, physicians prescribe a short course of a moderate dose of a corticosteroid drug called prednisone. If this is your liver specialist's approach, you may find that you are most pleasantly surprised by the effects of this anti-inflammatory medicine, which I'll talk about in more detail later on in this chapter. You may feel dramatically better and realize that although you thought you had no symptoms, in reality you had significant fatigue and malaise that abated or resolved completely with the treatment.

If your disease is more severe (that is, if you have pronounced elevations of the liver enzymes or gamma globulin levels, or both, and these levels remain high for a few months), *without treatment,* your risk of succumbing to autoimmune hepatitis is very high—up to 50 percent over the ensuing five-year period. Fortunately, however, 80 to 90 percent of patients with severe disease who receive treatment with corticosteroids have a favorable response to therapy.

COMPLICATIONS

One of the first questions that Janet asked me when I told her that she had autoimmune hepatitis was, "Am I going to get cirrhosis?" Although cirrhosis is a common complication of autoimmune hepatitis, Janet was fortunate in that she had no liver scarring.

She was also concerned that this condition might cause cancer. In over a quarter century of clinical practice, however, I've noted that one complication of cirrhosis—primary liver cancer, or hepatoma (cancer that arises within the liver, not cancer that originates elsewhere in the body and then spreads to the liver)—is singularly absent in patients with autoimmune hepatitis. In fact, I haven't seen a single case of this complication.

A short while ago when I gave a lecture on tumors of the liver at a Harvard postgraduate course, I polled an audience of approximately 400 U.S. gastroenterologists to see if anyone had seen primary liver cancer as a complication of autoimmune hepatitis. Not one individual in the audience raised his or her hand. Rare cases are mentioned in medical literature, but it's possible that some of these patients had other confounding factors (such as the newly discovered hepatitis C virus) that actually were causing their liver cancer.

TREATMENT

Like many patients who have been newly diagnosed with autoimmune hepatitis, Janet was very interested in her treatment options. She wondered, first of all, what those options were. And she wanted to know if she would be on medication for the rest of her life, or if she would ever need a liver transplant. Another question that came up when we were discussing her treatment was, "Is it safe to drink alcohol?"

Let me answer her last question first. If your liver biopsy shows that your autoimmune hepatitis is very mild, then alcohol consumption in small amounts is probably safe. A glass of wine or two on special occasions only—but not on a regular basis—should be fine. There are two exceptions, however. If you have viral hepatitis B or C infection—even a mild case—you should avoid alcohol altogether, because with these conditions this chemical works as an accelerator of liver injury. And if you have any form of *advanced* liver disease, it's best to avoid alcohol completely.

Drug Therapy

Prednisone, a form of corticosteroid, and a drug called azathioprine (Imuran), which may be given with prednisone, are lifesaving treatments for patients who have moderate to severe cases of autoimmune hepatitis.

The underlying immunological disorder in autoimmune hepatitis is not well understood. We do know that this disease involves defects in the regulation of the immune system; these defects facilitate the production of certain antibodies that can destroy liver cells. Corticosteroids and other immunosuppressive agents are of benefit, presumably because they can disrupt this destructive cell-damaging mechanism. Many people remain on this therapy for one to two years, and some need to continue to take medication indefinitely.

I prescribed prednisone for Janet, and she took it, in gradually reduced dosages, for about a year. Her recovery was swift and dramatic, with complete normalization of her liver function test results and total disappearance of her jaundice. Her fatigue and lack of appetite vanished, and she returned to full-time work. Two years after finishing the prednisone treatment, Janet continues to feel perfectly well.

SIDE EFFECTS OF PREDNISONE. Although corticosteroids such as prednisone can be lifesaving drugs, watch out for several side effects. If you take these medications, you should get regular eye exams to make sure that cataracts (clouding of the lenses of the eyes) have not developed. I also advise my patients who are taking corticosteroids on a long-term basis to see a specialist in metabolic bone disease for a test called bone densitometry every year to eighteen months; rarely, bone loss can occur. For that reason, I recommend 1,200 mg of supplemental calcium (in two doses per day) together with 1,000 international units of vitamin D every day. Other exciting new therapeutic options that show promise in preventing bone loss include drugs called Fosamax (alendronate), Miacalcin (which can be given as a nasal spray), and fluoride. Exercise such as walking, step aerobics, and working out on a treadmill also may be helpful in reducing bone loss.

Other side effects of corticosteroid therapy include glucose intolerance (a tendency to develop diabetes), impaired wound healing, and possibly an increased risk of developing infections.

SIDE EFFECTS OF IMURAN. If side effects of prednisone therapy alone present problems, your doctor may prescribe a lower dose of prednisone along with a "steroid-sparing" drug called Imuran. In general this drug is not used by itself, and it does not bring the autoimmune hepatitis into remission, but it can make lower doses of prednisone possible.

Imuran is a powerful immunosuppressant that also is given to patients after liver and other organ transplants to prevent their bodies from rejecting the new organ. For autoimmune hepatitis, however, much lower doses are given (100 to 150 mg/day). In such doses, Imuran acts not as an immunosuppressant but as an "immunomodulator"; in other words, this drug alters the immune system but does not suppress it.

Vast experience with the use of Imuran for autoimmune hepatitis shows that the risk of profound immunosuppression that can lead to certain malignancies (including lymphoma) is extremely low. Another significant but rare side effect of Imuran therapy is inflammation of the pancreas (pancreatitis), which can cause abdominal pain. In the unlikely chance that you do develop this side effect, you should notify your physician right away, because this drug will need to be discontinued.

EFFECTIVENESS. In general, your chance of survival is very good with treatment. One of my patients was a lady in her late twenties who had autoimmune hepatitis that had evolved into cirrhosis. She suffered from two major complications of cirrhosis: bleeding of the prominent veins (varices) in her esophagus and fluid buildup in her abdomen (ascites). She was on the waiting list for a liver transplant.

We treated her varices with an endoscopic procedure called variceal banding (the bleeding veins are tied off, or ligated, with a rubber-band-deploying device), and we got her ascites under control with diuretics and salt restriction. Prednisone suppressed her liver inflammation and indeed brought her condition into remission, so that her liver function test results became normal. Now, three years later, she is not taking any medication, she has had two beautiful children, and she is off the liver transplant list.

Like this patient, approximately 20 percent of people with autoimmune hepatitis can stay off their medication for months to years, although the risk of relapse remains. Other patients may need to continue drug therapy with moderate doses of prednisone and Imuran. Still others require a low-maintenance dose (2–5 mg/day) of prednisone for a long or indefinite period of time. Attempts to reduce their dosages can lead to a flare-up of the disease.

REMISSION AND RELAPSE. With corticosteroid therapy, chances are good that you will achieve remission, although you may experience a relapse of your disease months to years later. The occurrence of a relapse is totally unpredictable, so if your disease is in remission, you must seek immediate medical attention any time your symptoms reappear. These symptoms might include fatigue, nausea, arthralgia (joint pain), and dark urine. I also advise my patients to be examined by their primary care physician on at least an annual basis.

Cyclosporin A and FK-506

In the rare chance that the prednisone or Imuran fail to produce remission, your gastroenterologist may recommend that you see a hepatologist who has a great deal of experience in the treatment of autoimmune hepatitis. Such an expert may prescribe other medications such as cyclosporin A and a newer drug called FK-506. Both of these drugs are used as immunosuppressants following kidney and liver transplants.

LIVER TRANSPLANTS

An overwhelming majority of patients with autoimmune hepatitis will not require a liver transplant. However, if you do need one because you have severe disease involving cirrhosis and its complications (and medical therapy is unable to produce a remission), you should take solace and comfort in the fact that the five-year survival rate after a liver transplant for people with autoimmune hepatitis is greater than 80 to 90 percent. You also should be encouraged to know that this disease rarely recurs following this operation.

SUMMARY

Autoimmune hepatitis is an uncommon condition. It's generally not related to other autoimmune disorders, and it has no bona fide association with systemic lupus erythematosus (SLE). Other points to keep in mind if you have this condition are as follows:

- It's not contagious.
- The spectrum of liver injury encompasses very mild disease to severe disease with cirrhosis and its complications.
- If cirrhosis is present, you should be screened to see if you have esophageal varices. If you do have varices, you should take medication to decrease your risk of bleeding (see chapter 9).
- Even if you have cirrhosis along with your autoimmune hepatitis, your response to prednisone can be dramatic and lifesaving.

- One complication that is extremely rare—even in patients with cirrhosis—is the development of liver cancer (primary hepatocellular carcinoma).
- You most likely will not require a liver transplant, but if you do, you have an excellent prospect of survival, and the risk of recurrence of autoimmune hepatitis in your new liver is extremely low.
- If you have moderate to severe autoimmune hepatitis, you should not drink alcohol.

Research into what causes this condition and how it injures the liver is underway. Also, refinements of currently available treatments and the development of other forms of treatment are being explored actively in the United States and many other parts of the world.

8

Alcoholic Liver Disease

For dronkenesse is verray sepulture
Of mannes wit and his discrecioun.
—GEOFFREY CHAUCER, c. 1387

Alcohol is the great destroyer.
—JOHN HOGAN, 2000

From Chaucer to the great poet Milton, who long ago wrote of "the sweet poison of misused wine," people have long been aware of the consequences of drinking. Today we know that alcohol is indeed a sweet poison that can harm virtually every part of your body, including your heart, pancreas, and central nervous system. It is the progressive damage that alcohol does to your liver, however, that can create the most serious problems for your health.

How does alcohol "poison" your liver and put your health at risk? First of all, it can have a deleterious effect on your liver's ability to heal itself after it has been injured by other toxins, drugs, or viruses. It can also damage your liver more directly. When you drink, alcohol is absorbed rapidly from your stomach and intestines. Some of it travels to your lungs and kidneys, where it is excreted, but most of it is broken down and converted (metabolized) into other substances by your liver. A by-product of this complex metabolic process is a toxin called acetaldehyde. Acetaldehyde goes right to your liver cells, causing structural and functional changes that eventually can lead to alcoholic liver disease.

When doctors use the term *alcoholic liver disease,* they are referring to a specific disease process that is made up of four distinct, advancing stages of liver damage, beginning with something called fatty liver and, if unchecked, progressing to inflammation of the liver, or alcoholic hepatitis. The next, even more critical stage is severe liver scarring, or cirrhosis, which can sometimes result in liver cancer.

How prevalent is this problem? Alcoholism is the most common form of drug abuse in the United States and many other parts of the world. According to the U.S. National Institute on Alcohol Abuse and Alcoholism, approximately 11 million Americans consume five or six alcoholic drinks every day. (Each drink is approximately one can (12 oz.) of beer or ale; one glass (6 oz.) of wine; a small glass (4 oz.) of sherry, liqueur, or aperitif; or a single shot (1.5 oz.) of distilled 90-proof spirits.) Ten to 35 percent of these heavy drinkers will develop alcoholic hepatitis. Ten to 20 percent also will develop cirrhosis, and every year an estimated 10,000 to 24,000 people will die from it.

ARE YOU AT RISK?

Who are all of these heavy drinkers? You probably don't think of your neighbor as a drug abuser just because he often has a beer in his hand on weekends. After all, he has a good job and pays his mortgage every month—he doesn't exactly fit the "skid row" stereotype that may come to mind when we hear the word "alcoholic." In truth, very few alcoholics fit this down-and-out image. Alcoholism and its consequences can afflict persons from all walks of life, regardless of how old they are, where they came from, or how indigent or affluent they may be.

Throughout this chapter, you will find comments by my friend and colleague John Hogan, who is both a pathologist at the hospital where I work and a teacher of clinical medicine at a major university. When I first met John I had no idea that he had ever had, as he puts it, "a career as a drunk." Indeed, today he says that his professional accomplishments have far exceeded any of the "wildest expectations" that he may have had twenty-three years ago, when his primary goal in his working life was to make enough money to buy alcohol. Now when he looks back on his old "career," John reflects, "Alcohol is so confining."

Although alcoholics may be old or young, rich or poor, *susceptibility* to alcoholism and alcoholic liver disease is not as democratic. Imagine a crowded beach in the summertime. All of the individuals on that beach are being exposed to the same type of ultraviolet rays for about the same amount of time. Some will go home with a suntan, some will have a little sunburn, and some over the years will actually have the early stages of skin cancer. Likewise, if you went to a bar and every person there had two glasses of the same type of red wine, poured by the same bartender, not everyone would be affected by that wine in the same way. By extension, if the same people returned to that or another bar and consumed the same number of drinks every night for several months or years, not all would develop alcoholic liver disease.

GENETIC FACTORS

What makes some people more at risk for developing alcoholic liver disease than others? It might depend upon your genetic inheritance. Your risk is highest if you have an alcoholic (biological) parent, regardless of whether or not you grew up in that parent's home or were adopted by another family at birth. Having a sister or brother who is an alcoholic also increases your chances of developing alcoholic liver disease.

Researchers are trying to figure out which genes may make a person vulnerable to alcoholism, and some day in the not too distant future, screening may make it possible for high-risk individuals to receive early intervention and treatment. For now, though, if one of your parents is or was an alcoholic, you should be aware of your potential predisposition to this disease, and you should educate yourself and your family members about the dangers associated with drinking. If you're lucky, you won't have to concern yourself with this unfortunate inheritance at all. To the contrary, you may have a much more appealing birthright: you may have inherited genes that actually *protect* you from alcoholism.

Not long ago, researchers discovered that some Asians have just such a genetic makeup. They have low amounts of a certain enzyme that is critical for the metabolism of alcohol, and when they drink, the toxin that I mentioned earlier—acetaldehyde—accumulates quickly in their bodies and causes a "flushing reaction." This reaction, in turn, can lead to alcohol aversion.

I say this not to generalize or to imply that if you are Asian you are automatically immune from alcoholism and its consequences. This is simply a striking example of the role that genetics can play in a person's biologic response to alcohol.

GENDER

Your response to alcohol may also be affected by your gender. If a man and woman with the exact same body weight drink the same amount of alcohol, the woman will probably experience more severe liver injury. This is because after consuming alcohol, women have higher concentrations of alcohol per kilogram of body weight than men do. For the same reason, it takes less time for women to develop liver damage than it does for men. Women also appear to have a greater likelihood of developing alcoholic hepatitis and of dying from cirrhosis.

SETTING

In addition to your genes and gender, the setting in which you drink may be a strong determinant of whether or not you will develop an alcohol problem. For instance, a lot of college students get "smashed" fairly often, because college is believed by some to be a great place to drink! The average student has relatively few responsibilities. Most do not have a full-time job or children to attend to the morning after a big party.

Another one of my colleagues at Boston's Beth Israel Deaconess Medical Center, Dr. Adam Silk, is a psychiatrist who specializes in addictive disorders. He notes that "the cost-benefit of getting plastered is dramatically different" for college students than it is for most older adults. After college, most people do not drink as heavily as they did during their university years—and most do not become alcoholics—because their environment has changed. If the college life went on forever, though, many more people would have serious drinking problems. What a sobering thought! Likewise, a married husband and father who goes away for a weekend with his buddies to play golf may drink much more alcohol than he ordinarily would, but when he returns home and goes to his job on Monday morning, he probably won't take a six-pack of beer along with him, because he's no longer in a setting that's conducive to drinking.

For the same reason, although alcoholism is a huge problem among populations of homeless people, when individuals leave this environment and make a life for themselves off the street, their alcohol intake generally goes down.

Where do you drink alcohol? Who do you drink with? If you live or associate with friends or relatives who drink quite often, or if you are in a situation or environment that provides a lot of time to drink, you may have a greater chance of developing this addiction.

This is what happened to John Hogan:

> *I was an adult when I took my first drink on my twenty-first birthday, and I didn't particularly like it or dislike it, but I saw it as my passport into adulthood. I had the feeling that I was becoming a grown-up.*
>
> *Within a few years, I got myself into a group of heavy drinkers, and eventually I became a heavy drinker just like them. The funny part about it was that I found that I could drink barrels of the stuff and still be the one who drove everybody home. I had a great sense of pride that I was the one who had the "hollow leg." But in a two-year period, I went from being a social drinker to being a full-blown alcoholic.*

PSYCHOLOGICAL FACTORS

Your risk of drinking too much and developing alcoholic liver disease can also be related to your psychological health. By this I don't mean that you may have an "addictive personality." Such a thing may not even exist. But clearly there is a higher incidence of alcoholism among people whose psyches have been affected by illnesses such as manic-depression (also called bipolar disorder) and post-traumatic stress disorder (a psychological illness that may be triggered by an intensely disturbing experience such as rape or military combat) than among people who have not experienced these problems.

There appears to be a synergy between alcoholism and certain psychological conditions, too, so that if you're increasingly depressed, you may drink more than usual, and when you drink more than usual, you may become even more depressed.

CHRONIC HEPATITIS B AND C

Another factor that may affect your vulnerability to the destructive power of alcohol is chronic (or long-term) infection with either the hepatitis B or hepatitis C virus. If you have such an infection and you drink heavily, you have an increased chance of developing an advanced and potentially fatal liver disease such as cirrhosis. You also may experience liver damage at a younger age (and after drinking less alcohol) than you would otherwise.

You can turn back to chapters 3 through 6 for more information about both viruses and their other consequences. For now, though, keep in mind that if perchance you are infected with either hepatitis B or hepatitis C, drinking alcohol could be a formula for disaster.

OBESITY AND MALNUTRITION

In addition to the risk factors that I have described already, being obese for at least ten years may also heighten your susceptibility to alcoholic liver disease. At the other extreme, a diet of limited protein and carbohydrates may drain your liver of amino acids and enzymes and intensify alcohol's toxic effects, so malnutrition may make your liver disease more severe.

If you are overweight or undernourished, what should you do? Scientists currently are studying the way in which different diets may affect a person's response to alcohol, and in the near future, they may have some useful nutritional guidelines to offer. In the meantime, just be aware that good nutrition is important, and striving for a sensible weight is too. If you are grossly overweight or malnourished, know that alcohol consumption can be particularly bad for you.

DEADLY AGENTS: VITAMIN A
AND ACETAMINOPHEN (TYLENOL)

A final, important risk factor that I'd like to mention involves two commonplace substances that can be deadly to people who drink a lot of alcohol: vitamin A and acetaminophen (Tylenol). If you are a heavy drinker, taking too much of either one may predispose you to liver injury, worsen your already existing disease, or in extreme cases, even kill you.

Your liver is the storage place for more than 90 percent of your body's supply of vitamin A, and because this vitamin is fat-soluble, it can remain in your body for long periods of time. A buildup of vitamin A, in combination with the metabolic changes brought about by alcohol, can have a harmful effect on your liver function. Thus, if you drink alcohol, you should not consume more than the recommended daily allowance (or RDA) of vitamin A. For adults, that amount is 800 to 1,000 micrograms, or 4,000 to 5,000 international units per day. Most multivitamin pills contain 5,000 international units of this vitamin, so you could put yourself at risk simply by forgetting that you've already taken a multivitamin pill and taking another one in the same day. In general you need to be less concerned about ingesting too much vitamin A from ordinary foods.

If you drink alcohol regularly, you also should be extremely careful about taking acetaminophen (Tylenol). This is because if you drink heavily, your liver is "revved up" to convert, or metabolize, acetaminophen to large amounts of a particular toxin. In addition, if you are malnourished because of your drinking, you may not have enough of a certain enzyme that could help your body eliminate this toxin. Thus, if your metabolic system has been altered by alcohol, taking Tylenol can have severe consequences—*even if you only take it in amounts that would be safe and therapeutic for a healthy person who doesn't drink.* As few as six extra-strength Tylenol tablets or capsules (a total of 3 grams) taken all at once or taken over a very short period of time could lead to potentially fatal liver injury if you are a heavy drinker. In contrast, a person who doesn't consume a lot of alcohol would have to take an overdose of twenty extra-strength tablets or capsules (a total of 10 grams) to incur the same type of extreme liver damage.

Of course, if you have alcoholic liver disease, you shouldn't drink alcohol at all, but if you cannot or will not stop drinking, *don't take any more than four extra-strength Tylenol tablets or capsules (a total of 2 grams) in a twenty-four-hour period.* This same warning applies to other medications that contain acetaminophen. Table 8-1 lists many of them. Take a minute to go through this table—you'll likely be surprised at the number of common medications that contain this ingredient. Be especially careful when buying over-the-counter analgesic and fever-reducing products that contain acetaminophen, because some pediatric preparations (especially the liquid forms) contain different amounts or concentrations of this drug than the adult forms do. Also, many different brands of these products are available, and several look similar, so make sure that you don't accidentally substitute one for the other.

To help remind people that alcohol and acetaminophen can be a deadly combination, the U.S. Food and Drug Administration (FDA) recently announced that all over-the-counter pain relievers and fever reducers must carry a warning label advising people who consume three or more alcoholic drinks every day to consult their doctors before using these drugs. As I said earlier, though, the way in which your body responds to alcohol (and hence to agents like acetaminophen) depends on many different factors, including your weight and gender. Thus, if you are a woman of slight build who consumes two or three drinks per day, it may not be safe for you to take acetaminophen without seeking your doctor's advice first.

If you already have liver disease, you also should be cautious about taking other well-known pain relievers such as aspirin and nonsteroidal anti-inflammatory agents (NSAIDs) such as ibuprofen (Motrin, Advil), naproxyn sodium (Aleve), and ketoprofen (Orudis KT and Actron). These "blood-thinning" drugs affect the function of blood platelets, which are integral to the blood-clotting process. This alteration in your body's ability to control bleeding may be dangerous if you have certain complications of cirrhosis such as an increased bleeding tendency or engorged veins called varices in your esophagus that could rupture and bleed (see chapter 9).

If all of these pain relievers—acetaminophen, aspirin, and NSAIDs—may be harmful if you drink a lot of alcohol or if you have a bleeding

TABLE 8-1

Common Medicines that Contain Acetaminophen

Generic name	Trade (brand) name
acetaminophen	Acephen, Aceta, Acetaminophen Uniserts, Aminophen, Feverall, Genepap, Neopap, Panadol, Panex, Phenaphen, Suppap, Tenol, Tylenol, Valadol, Valorin
acetaminophen + butalbital	Axocet, Bancap, Bucet, Forte, Phrenilin, Sedapap, Tencon, Triaprin
acetaminophen + butalbital + caffeine	Anolor-300, Anoquan, Arcet, Axocet, Butace, Dolmar, Endolor, Esgic, Ezol, Femcet, Fioricet, Isocet, Isopap, Medigesic, Pacaps, Pharmgesic, Phrenilin, Repan, Tencet, Triad, Two-dyne
acetaminophen + butalbital + caffeine + codeine	Fioricet with codeine
acetaminophen + caffeine	Actamin, Aspirin-free Excedrin, Summit
acetaminophen + codeine + caffeine	Codalan
acetaminophen + codeine	Aceta with codeine, Acetaco, Capital with codeine, Empracet with codeine, Myapap with codeine, Phenaphen with codeine, Proval, Tylaprin with codeine, Tylenol with codeine, Ty-Pap with codeine, Ty-Tab with codeine
acetaminophen + hydrocodone	Anexsia, Anodynos-DHC, Bancap HC, Co-Gesic, Dolacet, DuoCet, Hycopap, Hydrocet, Hydrogesic, Hy-Phen, Lorcet, Lorcet Plus, Lortab, Margesic, Medipain, Norcet, Polygesic, Stagesic, T-Gesic, Vicodin, Vicodin ES, Vicodin-HP
acetaminophen + meperidine	Demerol APAP
acetaminophen + oxycodone	Endocet, Percocet, Roxicet, Roxilox, Tylox
acetaminophen + pentazocine	Talacen
acetaminophen + propoxyphene	Darvocet-N, Dolene AP-65, E-Lor, Propacet, Wygesic

tendency because of liver disease, what can you do for pain? I advise my patients to try heating pads, acupuncture, and, for the relief of chronic discomfort, the expertise of a pain management specialist.

STAGES OF ALCOHOLIC LIVER DISEASE

Now you know how various risk factors can affect the way in which your body responds to alcohol. If you *are* adversely affected by this "poison," you may have developed a very mild or a very severe case of alcoholic liver disease—or something in between. As I said earlier, alcohol-induced liver injury occurs in sequential stages. These include an early phase called fatty liver, followed by alcoholic hepatitis, alcoholic cirrhosis, and, in the most extreme cases, liver cancer.

FATTY LIVER

I'd like to tell you about a patient of mine who had the most mild form of alcoholic liver disease. Not long ago, a forty-eight-year-old woman named Lynda came to my office after she was referred to me for evaluation by her primary care physician. When her doctor had examined her, he found that everything was normal except that her liver was slightly enlarged. His concern that she might have some type of liver injury was confirmed by abnormal results on blood tests called liver function tests (LFTs). An ultrasound test also verified that her liver was mildly enlarged. When her doctor asked, Lynda said that she drank one or two glasses of wine once or twice every week. He continued to check her LFTs periodically, and when her LFTs remained abnormal over the next four months, he referred her to me for further evaluation.

When I first met Lynda and talked with her about her medical history, she told me, as she had told her primary care physician, that she was a "social drinker." I did a workup to look for common causes of liver dysfunction (such as chronic viral hepatitis and an iron overload disorder called hemochromatosis); all of these blood tests came back negative. I then performed a liver biopsy, which revealed a striking accumulation of fat within Lynda's liver. Under the microscope, her biopsy specimen presented a classic picture of fatty liver disease.

When Lynda came to see me a week later to go over the biopsy results, she was quite anxious about her diagnosis. She said, "Dr. Chopra, I feel well but I'm really worried. Do I have cirrhosis of the liver? What did the biopsy show?" I explained to Lynda that she did not have cirrhosis, but had developed a condition called fatty liver, which is the most common form of alcoholic liver disease. This condition could progress to cirrhosis. Once again I asked her about her drinking habits. She admitted that she actually had been consuming from three to four glasses of wine every day for the last several years. On occasion she would drink even more. She started to cry as she asked, "Have I caused irreparable damage to my liver? I'm too young to have liver disease. I have two little kids!"

I reassured Lynda that the damage that had been done was not irreparable. In fact, given the amount of alcohol that she had been drinking, she was actually quite lucky that her liver disease was still in this early, reversible stage. Generally even short-term consumption of small amounts of alcohol can lead to the same kind of mild liver damage with which Lynda was diagnosed.

Symptoms

If you, like Lynda, have fatty liver, you most likely won't have any symptoms. In fact, many people never even know that they have fatty liver disease. If you do experience symptoms, you may have a diminished appetite, mild nausea, vomiting, or minor abdominal pain.

Diagnosis

PHYSICAL EXAMINATION. You may go to your primary care physician because of these symptoms, or for another health problem altogether. When your doctor examines you, he or she may find that your liver is enlarged and possibly tender.

BLOOD TESTS. As part of your examination, your doctor probably will order a series of common blood tests, including liver function tests, or

LFTs. (These tests are explained in detail in chapter 2.) If the results of these tests show slight abnormalities, your physician may ask you about any drugs or herbal medications that you might be taking, since those could be responsible for abnormal LFTs. He or she almost certainly will talk with you about your alcohol consumption and may tell you that you need to stop drinking. You then will have to repeat the blood tests in a few months to see if there is any improvement.

If the results of your LFTs remain abnormal, your doctor probably will order another battery of tests to make sure that you don't have any other common liver disorders before referring you to a gastroenterologist (a doctor who specializes in disorders of the gastrointestinal system) or a hepatologist (a doctor who specializes in disorders of the liver).

RADIOLOGIC STUDIES AND LIVER BIOPSY. Your physician or specialist may then do further testing, including radiologic imaging studies such as an ultrasound scan and a procedure called a liver biopsy, which usually is done on an outpatient basis. (See chapter 2 for information on how this procedure is done and how you can prepare for it.) The biopsy can confirm the diagnosis of alcoholic liver disease and will help your doctor determine which stage of this disease you have. You may, for example, have fatty liver, or you may have a mild case of the next stage of alcoholic liver disease, which is called alcoholic hepatitis.

TESTS TO EXCLUDE OTHER CAUSES. In addition to ascertaining the nature and severity of your liver disease, appropriate testing is necessary to determine its exact cause. That's because even if you are a heavy drinker, something else may be responsible for your liver disorder. One potential cause is chronic infection with the hepatitis B or C virus. A simple blood test will show whether or not you are infected with one or both of these viruses. A blood test can also be done to exclude previous exposure to the hepatitis A virus.

If you don't have immunity against the hepatitis A and B viruses, your doctor probably will want to make sure that you receive both the HAV and HBV vaccines. That's because infection with either of these viruses, on top of your already existing liver disease, could make you very ill. (A vaccine directed against the hepatitis C virus is not yet available.) In addition to alcohol and viral hepatitis B and C, other causes of fatty liver include severe protein malnutrition or starvation, or the opposite problem—obesity; diabetes; and treatment with certain medications, including a corticosteroid drug called prednisone. Note that although in some instances prednisone can lead to fatty liver, it can be a lifesaving treatment for people with other liver disorders such as severe alcoholic hepatitis and autoimmune hepatitis.

Treatment

If, like Lynda's, your alcoholic fatty liver has not yet progressed to alcoholic hepatitis or cirrhosis, your prognosis is excellent, and your treatment is straightforward: you need to stop drinking alcohol, and you need to make certain that you have adequate nutrition. Most people who do so will completely recover.

However, if you have fatty liver, you'll have a high risk of developing more severe stages of liver injury, including full-fledged cirrhosis, if you continue to consume alcohol. A recent study from England described eighty-eight patients who had fatty liver disease for approximately ten years. Sixteen of these patients developed scar tissue (fibrosis), and some developed more significant scarring, or cirrhosis of the liver. Of these sixteen patients, fifteen had continued to drink alcohol.

If, in spite of your diagnosis of fatty liver, you are unsure about whether or not you have a true alcohol problem, I recommend that you answer the "CAGE" questions:

- Have you felt the need to **C**ut down on drinking?
- Have you ever felt **A**nnoyed by criticism of your drinking?
- Have you had **G**uilty feelings about drinking?
- Do you ever take a morning **E**ye opener (a drink first thing in the morning to steady your nerves or get rid of a hangover)?

Almost all alcoholics will answer yes to at least two of these questions, and approximately half will answer yes to all four questions. In contrast, most nonalcoholics will answer no to more than two questions, and more than 80 percent will answer no to all four questions.

If you answer the CAGE questions, the results may really surprise you. Granted, you may drink more than you should, but like many people, you may wonder how you could possibly have an alcohol problem that's severe enough to cause liver disease if you've never been drunk in your life! The truth is that drinking—not drunkenness—damages the liver. Even if you've never been intoxicated or have never missed a day of work because of your drinking, you can develop alcoholic liver disease if you've been consuming alcohol heavily for many years.

Another thing that people tend to wonder about is whether or not you can protect yourself from further liver damage if you stop drinking one type of alcoholic beverage and substitute another for it. In fact, the type of alcoholic beverage that you consume is unimportant—it's the alcohol *content* that counts. The liver, despite being one of the "smartest" organs in the body, cannot discriminate among beer, wine, and single-malt scotch; they all can be equally toxic.

> For the longest time, alcohol didn't mean that much to me. But alcohol is a very insidious thing. It slowly creeps into your body and starts to "own" you. It wasn't long before I began to lose everything, including my job and my self-respect. I got my first drunk driving violation. My life became totally unmanageable.
>   . . . Real alcoholism is this: you can't stop drinking when you start. You may promise yourself that you'll never do it again because you're so ashamed and you've hurt so many people, but it all goes out the window when that strange little button in your head gets clicked on. And you automatically try to justify everything just to have a drink. In my years of sobriety I've realized that everything I did while I was a drunk was done to protect my right to drink.
>
>   —JOHN HOGAN

Continuing to drink is especially dangerous if you have chronic hepatitis C virus infection, because alcohol is the most important "accelerator" of liver injury in people with this condition. I tell my patients to remember that they have two eyes, two lungs, and two kidneys—but only one liver. We don't want to chance causing irreparable damage to this vital organ. Therefore, if you have liver disease, total abstinence from alcohol is very important.

Once when I was talking with John Hogan about how he eventually stopped drinking, he told me that after years of trying to give up alcohol, he realized that this was an "all or nothing" commitment. He noted, "Once you've crossed the fine line from being a 'social drinker' to being an alcoholic, you can never go back to being just a social drinker again." Then he added this analogy: "If you take a cucumber and put it into brine, it will become a pickle. It may be the same shape and size as it was before, and it may still be green, but it will never be just a cucumber again."

Although it's easy to give such advice, I know that relinquishing this addictive habit can be very difficult. A little later on in this chapter, I'll talk more about how John succeeded in conquering this addiction and about different approaches to doing so. First, though, I'd like to tell you about another one of my patients who had the next stage of alcoholic liver disease—alcoholic hepatitis.

ALCOHOLIC HEPATITIS

Tom was a forty-three-year-old innkeeper from Vermont who went to see his primary care doctor at the insistence of his sister, who had been concerned that he looked pale and unwell. His doctor noticed immediately that Tom did look ill: his skin and the whites of his eyes had a yellowish hue (this is called jaundice), and he had a swollen, distended abdomen. He examined Tom and found that he had a tender, enlarged liver, an enlarged spleen, and a low-grade fever. He then did some bloodwork that confirmed that Tom had jaundice as well as anemia. His LFTs also showed some significant abnormalities. When asked about his drinking, Tom told his doctor that he used to drink one or two beers every day, but since the death of his wife in a tragic car accident the year before, he had been drinking more heavily.

Tom was admitted to the local hospital with a diagnosis of alcoholic hepatitis. His primary care physician requested that a gastroenterologist be consulted to help with Tom's treatment. The gastroenterologist concurred with the clinical diagnosis and suggested that a liver biopsy be performed. At this point, at the request of his sister, Tom was transferred to Boston's Beth Israel Deaconess Medical Center and was placed under my care.

When I met Tom and his sister shortly after he was admitted, they both had many questions about Tom's disease and his prognosis. I explained to them that alcoholic hepatitis refers to a distinct clinical syndrome that may develop after many years of heavy drinking. Just like hepatitis that is caused by viruses or certain autoimmune problems, in alcoholic hepatitis there is liver inflammation that can lead to liver scarring, or cirrhosis. The next day we performed a liver biopsy that confirmed that Tom indeed had both alcoholic hepatitis and cirrhosis.

Symptoms

Just as with fatty liver, if you have alcoholic hepatitis you may have no symptoms at all and may only learn of the disease because of unusual findings during a routine physical examination or because of abnormal findings on liver function blood tests. It's also possible that you might not have any of the common indications of this illness: fever (usually of less than 101°), fatigue, loss of appetite, nausea, weight loss, weakness, diarrhea, dark urine, light-colored stools, or jaundice. If you have a severe case of alcoholic hepatitis, you may be gravely ill with a fever as high as 104° that may last for several days to several weeks.

If you have alcoholic hepatitis and you continue to drink alcohol, or if your alcoholic hepatitis is diagnosed in its advanced stages, your disease can progress to cirrhosis, and there can be dire complications. They include:

- A tendency to have nosebleeds, bleeding gums, or even internal bleeding (this is because your liver is not producing blood clotting factors correctly)
- Fluid retention in the abdomen (this is called ascites—pronounced "a-SITE-ease"; see pages 164–67)
- Infection of the fluid that has built up in your abdomen (this is called "spontaneous bacterial peritonitis")

- Mental confusion, the hallmark of a syndrome called hepatic encephalopathy. This complication occurs when the poorly functioning liver fails to rid the body of toxins such as ammonia. An accumulation of these toxins can affect the central nervous system, causing sleepiness, disorientation, and sometimes coma. The treatment of hepatic encephalopathy is described on pages 170–71.
- Kidney failure related to severe liver scarring, or cirrhosis

People with *severe* alcoholic hepatitis have a 50 to 75 percent risk of dying from this disease if they receive no treatment. This high death rate exceeds by far the death rate from a heart attack.

Diagnosis

PHYSICAL EXAMINATION.   In addition to the symptoms described above, when your doctor examines you, he or she may find certain medical signs that are indicative of alcoholic hepatitis. For instance, you may have a tender, enlarged liver and spleen and enlarged parotid glands, as well as bruises on your skin caused by an increased bleeding tendency.

Other classic signs of chronic liver disease are spiderlike blood vessels at the surface of the skin (these are called spider nevi, or telangiectasias) and red palms. These signs, which are sometimes present in normal pregnancy, have long been associated with alcohol abuse. In the late 1950s, Dr. William Bennett Bean wrote the following limerick as a reminder of this relationship:

> *An older Miss Muffett*
> *Decided to rough it*
> *And lived upon whiskey and gin.*
> *Red hands and a spider*
> *Developed outside her—*
> *Such are the wages of sin.*

LABORATORY TESTS.   Alcohol also affects your bone marrow's production of infection fighters, or white blood cells. If you have alcoholic hepatitis, laboratory tests may show that you have a low white blood cell count; this may be the case if alcohol is preventing your bone marrow from doing its job or if your enlarged spleen is "hoarding" white cells. Damage to your bone marrow, as well as other problems such as gastrointestinal blood loss and a deficiency of folic acid, may cause you to develop a reduced red blood cell count, or anemia.

If your liver is severely inflamed, it's also possible that you may have an elevated, rather than a decreased, white blood cell count. The degree of this elevation will most likely correspond to the severity of your liver damage. If you have an extreme case of liver inflammation, your white blood cell count may be elevated to such a level that it rivals that of people who have leukemia. This "leukemoid reaction" explains why some doctors may initially suspect leukemia instead of alcoholic liver disease. In any case, it's imperative for your doctor to make sure that your high white blood cell count is not related to another cause such as infection. When your liver inflammation begins to subside, this count should go down as well.

Two other blood test results that may be high if you have moderate or severe alcoholic hepatitis are serum bilirubin and prothrombin time (PT). Bilirubin is a pigment that builds up in your body if you have liver disease. It can stain your skin, leading to a condition that is sometimes called "yellow jaundice." PT is a measure of your liver's ability to synthesize blood clotting factors. If your bilirubin and PT results are markedly abnormal, you could have severe alcoholic hepatitis and, if it is untreated, a 50 to 75 percent chance of dying from it.

Kidney function is usually normal in people with mild alcoholic hepatitis. To make sure that your kidneys have not been affected by your liver disease, though, your doctor will perform two blood tests called blood urea nitrogen (BUN) and creatinine. If these levels are elevated, you may be developing hepatorenal syndrome, a very serious disorder in which there is kidney failure due to a severe liver condition. Liver transplants are the only known solution for this syndrome, which is described in greater detail on page 172.

LIVER BIOPSY. As with all types of liver disease, the most definitive way of diagnosing alcoholic hepatitis is by performing a liver biopsy. In addition to its diagnostic value, a liver biopsy is useful for confirming the stage or degree of your liver disease and for excluding other factors that may be causing your LFTs to be abnormal. However, if your liver

Dr. Maddrey's Formula

Your gastroenterologist or hepatologist may use something called "Dr. Maddrey's discriminant function or formula" to determine the severity of your alcoholic hepatitis. In this formula, your prothrombin time (PT) is measured in seconds, and the "control" (normal) PT measurement is subtracted from it. The resulting number then is multiplied by 4.6 and added to your serum bilirubin level (in milligrams per deciliter). If the resulting number is greater than or equal to 32, your prognosis will be poor *without treatment*.

When I examined my patient Tom in the hospital, I found that he had jaundice, an enlarged liver and spleen, prominent "spider" veins, and red palms. The results of two of his laboratory blood tests were:

- Serum total bilirubin = 12 mg/dl (normal is < 1 mg/dl)
- PT = 19 seconds (normal is 13 seconds)

Using the formula outlined above, taking Tom's PT time of 19 seconds minus the normal control PT time of 13 seconds = 6. 6 x 4.6 = 27.6. If we add to this number Tom's serum bilirubin count (12), the result would be 39.6. Thus, my patient had severe alcoholic hepatitis (the "discriminant function" was greater than 32), and his prognosis—without treatment—would have been very poor.

disease is very advanced, a liver biopsy can be dangerous because of the potential for serious bleeding. In this case, your doctor may make the clinical diagnosis without performing a liver biopsy.

Chapter 2 describes the different types of liver biopsies and provides guidelines for how you can prepare for this type of procedure. The results of a liver biopsy, which is usually done on an outpatient basis, are generally available in a day or two. Your physician can help you to interpret the pathologist's report. You may want to have the following list of questions in hand when you are discussing these results with your doctor:

- Did my liver biopsy show features of alcoholic hepatitis? (These features might include distorted and dying liver cells, as well as infiltration of the liver cells with fatty deposits and white blood cells.)
- Were there increased amounts of iron in the liver (these iron deposits may be the sign of an iron overload disorder known as hemochromatosis; see chapter 11), abnormal deposits of copper in

the liver (Wilson's disease, see page 158), or features of infection with the hepatitis C virus?

- Did my liver biopsy show evidence of substantial scar tissue that would indicate that my disease has progressed to cirrhosis?

ENDOSCOPY. If your liver biopsy did reveal that you have alcoholic cirrhosis, your hepatologist or gastroenterologist will recommend that you undergo a procedure called an endoscopy to look for engorged veins (varices) in your esophagus. Varices are a serious consequence of liver disease because ruptured varices can result in severe and potentially fatal bleeding.

An endoscopy is a very simple test with an extremely low complication rate. Information about how you can prepare for this procedure is provided in the next chapter (chapter 9). If you undergo an endoscopy and your doctor finds that you do have varices, he or she may prescribe a drug called Inderal (propanolol). This drug, which is also used to treat high blood pressure, or hypertension, will decrease your risk of bleeding from these engorged veins.

Treatment

If your doctor determines that you have alcoholic hepatitis, you will be admitted to the hospital so that you can get enough bed rest, stay away from alcohol, and eat a nutritious diet supplemented with appropriate vitamins. In the hospital, an anti-inflammatory drug called prednisone may be administered, and the doctors and nurses also will be able to monitor your condition carefully and treat you for any complications that may arise.

ALCOHOL COUNSELING

At this time, your physician probably will discuss with you and your family the ramifications of this disease process and the consequences that may befall you if you continue to drink alcohol.

If your doctor tells you that you must stop drinking, how can you begin to approach this enormous challenge? Today three main avenues are available: inpatient counseling, outpatient counseling, and self-help groups such as Alcoholics Anonymous. Let's look at these different options.

INPATIENT COUNSELING. While you're in the hospital, your internist may provide you with alcohol counseling, or he or she may give you a referral to speak with a social worker or a psychiatrist. Depending on the severity of your alcohol addiction, you also may qualify for an organized inpatient alcohol recovery program.

Until about five to eight years ago, the standard inpatient alcohol recovery program lasted twenty-eight days. This "Minnesota model" of treatment provided medicine to control the symptoms of alcohol withdrawal, individual counseling, and group therapy or Alcoholics Anonymous (AA) meetings. Today managed care has changed all of that. Insurance companies did not want to pay for such long-term care, so now they may cover only brief inpatient "detoxification" if your doctor determines that you will go into withdrawal if you stop consuming alcohol.

Some people do develop a physiological dependence syndrome that causes them to experience something like heroin withdrawal when they stop drinking. However, many binge drinkers (people who occasionally overindulge but can still get to work every day) do not develop withdrawal symptoms, so it may be difficult, if you are this kind of drinker, for you to get into an inpatient treatment program.

Today the fewest patients—those who suffer from the most severe alcohol impairment—receive the most resources. If you do qualify for such a program, you may receive as little as three to five days of inpatient care at an addiction treatment unit of a general or psychiatric hospital. During this time, you may be given tranquilizers called benzodiazepines to prevent or ease symptoms of alcohol withdrawal such as delirium tremens (d.t.'s), or "trembling delirium." Commonly used benzodiazepines include diazepam (Valium); chlordiazepoxide (Librium); and lorazepam (Ativan).

If you have severe alcoholic hepatitis with or without cirrhosis and these sedatives are absolutely needed to relieve the effects of alcohol withdrawal, the lowest possible dose should be taken. That's because these medications can precipitate or trigger a serious complication known as hepatic encephalopathy, an alteration in consciousness ranging from mild mental confusion to frank coma. For this reason, physicians sometimes choose to administer sedatives such as Ativan that are not metabolized (broken down) by the liver.

Other drugs that sometimes are used in the treatment of alcohol addiction include disulfiram (Antabuse) and naltrexone (Revia). Antabuse, which first was introduced to clinical use in the late 1940s, causes a very unpleasant reaction when patients consume even small amounts of alcohol. This preventive therapy is intended to make it harder to drink impulsively. Does it work? A rigorous controlled trial with this drug was reported in 1986. Researchers noted that patients who took Antabuse drank alcohol less frequently than they had before taking it, but the Antabuse did not prolong the time until the patient began drinking again, nor did it improve overall rates of abstinence from alcohol consumption. Notably, there was a low rate of compliance among this group of patients (that is, many of the patients did not follow the prescribed drug regimen), probably because of fear of the negative side effects (flushing, throbbing headache, nausea, vomiting, and sweating) that can occur after taking Antabuse and drinking alcohol. The other negative aspect of this drug is that, rarely, it has been associated with cases of acute and severe liver inflammation, or hepatitis.

In spite of these downsides, Antabuse may be an effective therapeutic adjunct when given to patients under daily and direct supervision. This view is validated by a study that showed that monitored use of this drug reduced patients' alcohol consumption over a six-month period.

In recent years, in addition to appreciating the importance of genetics and psychosocial aspects in the development of addictions, researchers have recognized the role of specific neurochemical changes in the brain that occur in people with alcoholism and other addictive disorders. Dr. Alan Leshner, director of the National Institute of Drug Abuse, has defined addiction as "not simply a lot of drug or alcohol use but a disease of the brain that is expressed as behavior and influenced by the social context in which it was developed." In other words, alcohol and other habit-forming substances considerably alter brain pathways and change the concentrations of "chemical messengers" in the brain called neurotransmitters. These changes can persist long after a person stops using an addictive substance.

An understanding of this biological basis for addiction has led to better pharmacological approaches in the treatment of addictive disorders. For example, animal research has revealed that alcohol stimulates the release of narcoticlike "feel-good" substances in the brain; these substances are called endogenous opioids. Drugs that block the effects of these opioids thus should take away these biochemical rewards and in turn decrease a person's alcohol consumption. To block endogenous opioids, scientists have looked to drugs called antagonists, which "cancel out" the effects of other substances.

In 1992 two groups of investigators found that 50 mg daily of an opioid antagonist called naltrexone given over a three-month period resulted in less-frequent alcohol craving in humans. These individuals were less likely to relapse to heavy drinking, and when they did drink, the amount of total alcohol that they consumed was significantly less than the amount that they drank before they began taking naltrexone.

Naltrexone is now an FDA-approved drug for patients who are participating in an alcohol recovery program. Like disulfiramine, naltrexone has to be taken voluntarily by patients, but careful monitoring by physicians to ensure compliance is important. For the most part, this drug is well tolerated, although some side effects such as nausea, dizziness, headache, and nervousness have been known to occur. Another promising drug is acamprosate, an agent that seems to safely modify alcohol-drinking behavior, with the only side effect being diarrhea. Together with supportive psychotherapy, it has been shown to result in increased periods of abstinence from drinking.

In addition to drug therapy and counseling with specialists in the treatment of alcohol addiction, inpatient programs may rely heavily on self-help groups such as AA. Inpatient treatment usually occurs in a hospital, although a few free-standing centers for addictive disorders still exist. Because they are so expensive to run, however, they are becoming less and less common. You may be aware of a handful of famous treatment centers that cater mostly to the wealthy. Many of these programs, which are out of the financial reach of most Americans, require cash up front. In speaking with Dr. Silk, mentioned earlier in this chapter, I was surprised to learn that you literally may have to walk in the door with a check for $14,000 if you want to stay for a month at one of these facilities.

OUTPATIENT COUNSELING. Since managed care stopped paying for most twenty-eight-day programs, many "intensive outpatient programs" have sprung up. For this type of therapy, you will go to the hospital or treatment facility for four to five hours every day, five days a week, for three to six weeks. Like the inpatient alcohol recovery programs, outpatient programs provide alcohol counseling with specialists in addictive disorders, and they usually also incorporate self-help groups such as AA. Although these programs are much cheaper for insurers than inpatient programs (they don't involve the high overhead costs of a twenty-four-hour facility), they are still expensive to run, and several have had difficulty staying in business. There are thus fewer of these outpatient programs available than there were twenty-eight-day programs a decade ago.

You don't necessarily have to enroll in an intensive outpatient program to find support, however. Mental health professionals generally are trained in the treatment of addictive disorders, and many people find it helpful to talk with a psychiatrist, psychologist, psychiatric social worker, or psychiatric nurse.

SELF-HELP GROUPS. More than half of all heavy drinkers who seek alcohol counseling and support turn to their primary care physicians or to self-help groups like Alcoholics Anonymous. As I've just mentioned, "twelve-step" programs like AA are also important components of both inpatient and outpatient treatment programs.

My friend John Hogan cautions that participation in such a program does not guarantee an automatic cure for alcoholism. "We live in an 'instant' society of instant gourmet meals and instant replays," he says, "but there's no such thing as 'instant sobriety.' It takes a long time. Just because you take the drink out of a person's hand does not mean that he or she is going to get sober and well right away." John was very lucky in that, in spite of his many years of heavy drinking, he didn't develop severe liver disease. However, his liver definitely was affected by all of the alcohol that he consumed, and it wasn't until six years after he stopped drinking that the results of his liver function tests finally returned to normal!

John attended a twelve-step program off and on for years before he finally stopped drinking; for him, this process was less twelve steps ahead than it was two steps forward and two steps back. In the end, though, it was the support of others in this program, in his workplace, and in the community, rather than any medical solution, that saved his life:

> *At first I remember not wanting to go to a twelve-step program because I didn't want to hear about a "higher power." I didn't want to hear about religion.*
>
> *Now I find that concern ironic, because actually most alcoholics pray every day. We pray that the bar will open. We pray that we won't get thrown out. We pray that we left enough in the jug from the night before. We pray all the time!*
>
> *. . . From 1970 to 1976, I bounced in and out of a twelve-step program. I'd go to meetings for so many weeks, and then I'd go out and drink. I never stayed dry any more than thirteen or fifteen days. I couldn't. By the fifteenth day I was out of my mind. I had to have a drink.*
>
> *I can't tell you how many times I tried [to quit] during that period of time. And I kept going back to meetings. Finally, after many years of trying to stop drinking, I surrendered. It's either that or you die.*

If you are looking for support in your efforts to stop drinking, your physician, social worker, or mental health care counselor can provide you with information about the meeting time and place of the self-help group nearest you.

NUTRITIONAL COUNSELING

In addition to finding a good alcohol recovery program, it may be useful to see a nutritionist who can help you replenish your body's stores of nutrients that have been used up by years of drinking. Alcohol provides only empty calories, and if you drink too much you may take in as much as 30 to 50 percent of your total calories from alcohol, so you may be lacking in essential vitamins (such as thiamine and folate), minerals (such as phosphate and magnesium), and protein.

Also, if alcohol has damaged your pancreas, you may be malnourished because this organ can no longer produce enough digestive enzymes necessary for the proper assimilation of food. If this is the case, you may need to stay on a low-fat diet and take pancreatic enzyme capsules or tablets (this supplement is called pancrelipase, or Pancrease) to correct this imbalance.

DRUG THERAPY

If your doctor finds that you have a mild case of alcoholic hepatitis without cirrhosis, you have a low risk of dying from liver disease. Just as with fatty liver, if you do nothing more than abstain from alcohol, your liver injury can completely resolve—no drugs are needed. Earlier in this chapter, I described drugs that sometimes are used in inpatient treatment centers to ease the effects of alcohol withdrawal and to disrupt the biochemical lure of drinking again. But what about drugs to treat the liver damage that alcohol already has wrought?

If you have a severe case of alcoholic hepatitis (as determined by Dr. Maddrey's formula; see box, page 135), a short course of a corticosteroid such as prednisone may improve your prognosis. For alcoholic hepatitis, prednisone is administered in a hospital or treatment center. It works as an anti-inflammatory agent to reduce the significant liver damage that is associated with this condition.

While you are taking this type of medication, your doctor will have to monitor you carefully for the development of side effects. For example, corticosteroids can modulate the immune response and increase your susceptibility to infection, and if infection develops, your medical team may decide that you should discontinue this treatment. Even if you don't experience side effects and you continue to take prednisone, it may take several months for you to fully recover.

My patient Tom, mentioned earlier in this chapter, was treated with prednisone for one month, and he tolerated this medication well. His liver condition improved dramatically as the reversible component of his disease—the alcoholic hepatitis—abated. Unfortunately, the irreversible scar tissue that he had already developed before his diagnosis remains with him, and we have to monitor him carefully for potential complications. Tom is feeling well, though, and he has returned to work. We hope, along with his family, that he won't return to drinking.

LIVER TRANSPLANTATION

For people with advanced alcoholic liver disease (severe alcoholic hepatitis, cirrhosis, and/or liver cancer), liver transplants have a 60 to 70 percent success rate. However, liver transplantation for people with alcoholic liver disease has been hotly debated in medical circles and liver transplant centers: there are not enough livers available for donation, there are long waiting lists for transplants, and transplant procedures and the resulting long-term management of patients who have had these operations are very expensive. Health care providers sometimes question whether these scarce resources should be committed to people who have "brought their liver injury on themselves" by drinking alcohol.

Although medical students, nurses, and physicians seem to have compassion for people with other "self-inflicted" health problems such as chronic lung disease caused by smoking, in my experience they often have a different attitude toward alcoholics. I feel strongly that this bias is unfortunate and inappropriate. As I mentioned earlier, the most important precursor of alcoholism seems to be alcoholism in a biological parent. In a very true sense, if you have a problem with alcohol, you may have "inherited" it, and the deck may have been stacked against you from the outset. Also, many studies have shown that people with alcoholic liver disease who undergo liver transplantation can do well and have five-year survival rates similar to those of people who have received liver transplants for nonalcoholic liver disease. One study reviewed follow-up data on alcoholic patients who had liver transplants in the United States between 1988 and 1995. These researchers found that deaths of patients in this group were related not to alcohol but to the same conditions (for instance, infection, cancer, or heart disease) that caused the deaths of nonalcoholic patients.

So, if you have had a drinking problem (but you are not an active substance abuser), if you don't have any other significant diseases, and if you are able to abstain from alcohol for approximately three to six months, there is no moral, ethical, or medical reason to preclude you from consideration for liver transplantation.

If a liver transplant is in your future, turn to chapter 13 for further information about how this operation works and how you can prepare for it. Keep in mind that you will require strong family and social support to help you manage long-term care and likely lifelong immuno-suppressive drug therapy after surgery.

ALCOHOLIC CIRRHOSIS

After fatty liver disease and alcoholic hepatitis, alcoholic cirrhosis is the next stage in alcoholic liver disease. Cirrhosis of the liver has been a very common cause of death in people in the most productive years of their lives, between the ages of thirty-five and sixty years. Fortunately, though, a recent study from the National Hospital Discharge Survey showed that the incidence of deaths related to alcoholic cirrhosis is declining.

In many people with cirrhosis, alcohol plays an important causative role, either by itself or in concert with other factors such as infection with the hepatitis B or C virus or an "iron overload" disorder (such as hemochromatosis; see chapter 11). Like people with milder forms of alcoholic liver disease (fatty liver and alcoholic hepatitis), if you have alcoholic cirrhosis and you continue to drink alcohol, your prognosis will be much worse than it would be if you stopped drinking.

The next chapter (chapter 9) describes cirrhosis and its treatment in more detail.

PRIMARY LIVER CANCER

Primary liver cancer, which also is referred to as primary hepatocellular carcinoma or hepatoma, is the most severe stage of alcoholic liver disease, and your risk of developing it is highest if you are also infected with the hepatitis B virus or hepatitis C virus. The symptoms, diagnosis, and treatment of primary liver cancer are described fully in chapter 12.

RESEARCH AND HOPE FOR THE FUTURE

Given the prevalence and serious nature of alcoholic liver disease, intense efforts to understand how alcohol causes liver injury and to develop more effective treatments are being carried out in many research centers throughout the world. Some of the promising therapies that scientists currently are exploring include innovative nutritional supplements and a drug called pentoxifylline.

Nutritional Supplements

POLYUNSATURATED LECITHIN (PUL). Dr. Charles S. Lieber, director of the Alcohol Research and Treatment Center and Liver Disease and Nutrition Section of the Bronx Veterans Affairs Medical Center, has done elegant studies that show that a naturally occurring compound called polyunsaturated lecithin extract prevents the development of cirrhosis in baboons who have been fed alcohol. This substance, which also goes by the verbally challenging name polyenylphosphatidylcholine (or simply PPC), is a "supernutrient" derived from soybeans. In the future, this supernutrient may be found to be an important part of nutritional therapy for people with alcoholic liver disease.

REPLACEMENT OF SAMe. Dr. Lieber also has found that long-term alcohol ingestion in baboons depletes the liver of another naturally occurring "supernutrient": an amino acid called S-adenosyl-l-methionine (SAMe, or AdoMet). Administration of a synthetic preparation of this compound appears to lessen the liver injury due to alcohol in primates, so scientists are exploring the use of such supplements for humans with alcoholic liver disease. An exciting clinical trial with AdoMet was recently undertaken in a long-term, multicenter study involving patients with alcoholic cirrhosis. This study indicated that long-term administration of AdoMet supplements may improve the chance of survival and delay the need for liver transplantation in patients with alcoholic cirrhosis, particularly in those with less advanced liver disease. A noteworthy feature of this study was that the treatment was well tolerated, and there were no serious side effects due to AdoMet. Larger studies need to be done to validate these findings.

TNF Inhibition

Investigators also are exploring the use of an anti-inflammatory agent called pentoxifylline to inhibit a protein called tumor necrosis factor (TNF) in people with alcoholic liver disease.

TNF, a protein that certain cells create in response to poisonous substances called endotoxins, is present in large amounts in people with a variety of malignant and inflammatory disorders such as alcoholic hepatitis. These high levels of TNF may cause further liver damage in people with alcoholic liver disease, so inhibition of this protein with pentoxifylline may be beneficial. A pilot study with this agent has shown promise.

9

· ·

Cirrhosis

Jack is a forty-eight-year-old attorney who lives and works just outside of Boston. He and his wife, Cynthia, are happily married and working hard to put their two daughters through college. He's also health-conscious: he eats well, works out at a gym near his office, and runs five miles every day. You wouldn't know from his outward appearance that he dabbled with intravenous drugs and consumed a fair amount of alcohol in the 1970s.

A few months ago Jack went to see his internist, Dr. Robert Hyde, to get a physical examination for life insurance purposes. Dr. Hyde did some routine blood tests and found that Jack's liver function test results were abnormal. He then tested Jack's blood for the hepatitis C virus (HCV), and the result was positive—it appeared that he was infected with the virus. At that point, Dr. Hyde referred Jack to me for further testing and treatment. On the summer morning when Jack came to my office, he was still reeling from the news. "Is it possible that there could have been a mixup with those blood tests? I can't believe that I have hepatitis C!" he exclaimed.

I assured him that the blood tests that he had taken were likely accurate, but that we would be doing more tests to confirm that he was infected and to find out exactly how serious his illness was.

Then he continued, "I feel perfectly fine—wouldn't I feel sick or have jaundice if I really had hepatitis? I'm sure your tests will show that if I do have it, I don't have a very severe case."

After talking at length with Jack about his medical history and the tests that had been done already, I explained that hepatitis C can occur with no symptoms whatsoever, and this infection may have resulted from using a single contaminated needle when he was taking intravenous drugs decades ago. I then told him that I was glad that he didn't have symptoms, but his lack of symptoms didn't necessarily mean that he had a mild case of HCV infection—only a biopsy would reveal how much damage the virus had done to his liver. During the biopsy, which would be performed as an outpatient procedure, a very small piece of tissue would be taken from his liver and then examined under the microscope. I drew some blood tests to measure how many copies of the virus were circulating in his blood and to check which genetic strain, or genotype, of the virus he was infected with. We scheduled his liver biopsy for the following week.

When the results came back a few days after the biopsy, Jack returned to my office to talk about them. I had the unfortunate task of telling him that when the pathologist and I had viewed his liver biopsy specimen under the microscope, we saw that there was substantial connective tissue or scar tissue (in medical jargon, this is called fibrosis) that had caused severe distortion of the liver architecture. In other words, the viral hepatitis infection had indeed damaged Jack's liver—to the degree that it had produced the chronic, progressive disease called cirrhosis.

Jack was completely shocked. "But I'm not that old!" he said, "and I'm not an alcoholic! In fact, I haven't touched a drop of alcohol in seven years! I feel perfectly well, and now you're telling me that I have both hepatitis C *and* cirrhosis?"

Jack's reaction wasn't unusual. Many people mistakenly believe that cirrhosis affects mostly the elderly and alcoholics, when in fact this disease can affect people of all ages, and alcoholism is only one of its many causes. Of the several thousands of Americans who died from cirrhosis in 1996, half were younger than sixty, and less than half were alcohol abusers. Cirrhosis is also more common than one might think: that year it was the tenth leading cause of death in the United States.

Jack's absence of symptoms also wasn't unusual. Like hepatitis C, cirrhosis may be "silent," not causing any noticeable health problems.

Sometimes it's an unexpected finding during an operation involving the gallbladder, stomach, pancreas, or colon—and sometimes it's only discovered during an autopsy. We call this "subclinical disease," because it hasn't produced any major clinical consequences.

Jack continued to express his astonishment during our discussion, but I could sense that he was ready to talk about where we needed to go from here to manage his disease. He continued, "Since I got those test results back from Dr. Hyde's office, I've been reading everything I can find about hepatitis and the liver. One magazine article mentioned that the liver can heal itself. Does that mean that my hepatitis infection and cirrhosis eventually will go away if I continue to take care of myself and eat the right foods?"

I said that it's true that the liver can heal itself—sometimes. I shared with him the Greek myth about the giant named Prometheus, who stole fire from heaven and gave it to mankind. This act infuriated the gods, who chained Prometheus to a rock to punish him. To add to the giant's torture, every day a vulture swooped down and devoured part of his liver. At night, though, after the bird left, the liver grew back, and Prometheus survived. For centuries people have known about the regeneration of healthy liver tissue, which they have viewed as one of the miraculous wonders of life. Today we know that if one person donates part of her liver to another person who needs a liver transplant, the donor's liver will regenerate within a few weeks. We also know that people who experience sudden acute liver failure because of viruses, drugs, or toxins occasionally can recover on their own as the liver regenerates and becomes perfectly normal (Figure 9-1).

Unfortunately for Jack, though, with cirrhosis this regenerative process fails to produce magic and may in fact be detrimental. Damaged liver cells are replaced not by healthy new cells but by scar tissue that interferes with the flow of blood through this important organ. As the liver architecture becomes distorted, the liver may no longer function normally (Figure 9-2).

Jack was clearly disappointed with this answer. "Well, if my liver can't heal itself, are there any drugs that will help?" he asked.

I explained that there is no single "magic bullet" to treat cirrhosis. In fact, this extensive scarring of the liver generally isn't reversible. The best we can do is to limit any further damage by managing the underlying disease that caused the cirrhosis in the first place.

The different therapies that are available thus vary widely depending on what caused the cirrhosis and on which (if any) complications have developed. That's why a careful diagnosis is so critical. If you, like Jack, have been diagnosed with cirrhosis, it will be very important for you to find a specialist who is experienced in managing problems of the gastrointestinal system (a gastroenterologist) or the liver (a hepatologist). While determining your best course of treatment, such specialists should be able to answer the following questions:

- Do you really have cirrhosis?
- If so, how severe is your disease?
- What caused your cirrhosis?
- Does the cause of your cirrhosis have any important ramifications for your family?
- Have you had any complications from your cirrhosis? What is your risk for developing complications in the years to come?
- What treatments are available for the condition that caused your liver scarring?

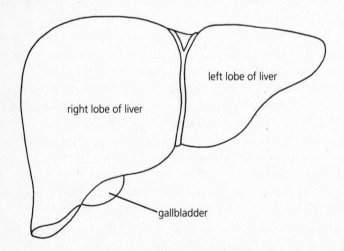

Figure 9-1. The Healthy Liver

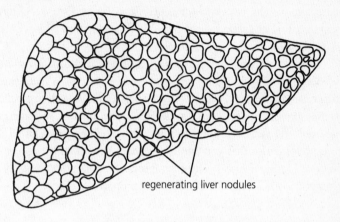

regenerating liver nodules

Figure 9.2. The Cirrhotic Liver

Let's talk about the steps that your gastroenterologist or hepatologist might take to answer these questions. I'll start by going over the symptoms that you might have with cirrhosis, and then explain how doctors diagnose and assess the severity of your disease. Next I'll tell you about the many causes of cirrhosis and how these causative factors can affect your treatment and your family. Finally, I'll discuss the complications of cirrhosis and the various therapies available for them.

DO YOU REALLY HAVE CIRRHOSIS?

SYMPTOMS

I got very sick the day after my thirty-fifth birthday. From there it snowballed, and I got sicker and sicker. I had a constant upset stomach, but I didn't feel all that weak. It was just a really nauseous feeling all the time, and I lost my appetite. It was like having the flu, and yet there were some good days when you wouldn't think that there was anything wrong with me.

In the early stages of cirrhosis, you may, like Jack, have no symptoms, or you may have vague symptoms such as fatigue, nausea, loss of appetite, and weight loss. Sometimes people with this disease also have itchy skin, jaundice (yellow discoloration of the skin and whites of the eyes), or increased sensitivity to drugs.

If you are a woman and you have advanced cirrhosis, hormonal imbalances may disrupt your ovulation cycle. If you are a man, these imbalances may cause your breasts to grow large (this condition is called gynecomastia) or your testes to shrink, or atrophy. You also may tend to bruise or bleed easily, have shortness of breath, and begin to retain fluid in your abdomen so that you appear pregnant (this is called ascites—pronounced "a-SITE-ease"). These symptoms are linked to some complications of cirrhosis that I'll talk about later on in this chapter.

DIAGNOSIS

Like Jack, many people who have no symptoms of cirrhosis only discover that they have this liver disease when they visit their primary care physician for other medical conditions or for an annual physical examination. Other people seek medical attention because they're experiencing some of the symptoms that I've just described. Still others first go to a doctor when their cirrhosis already is fairly advanced and they have complications such as breathing problems, bleeding, or ascites.

PHYSICAL EXAMINATION AND BLOOD TESTS. Your doctor's suspicion of cirrhosis may be raised during your physical examination if he or she finds that you have an enlarged spleen. Your liver itself may be normal in size, enlarged, or shrunken.

Abnormal results of certain common blood tests called liver function tests (LFTs) provide another clue. If these results are not normal, your doctor may have you repeat this battery of blood tests before referring you to a gastroenterologist or hepatologist with a recommendation that you undergo a liver biopsy.

> *I went to my family doctor, and he checked my liver function tests. My numbers would fluctuate. They'd go up and they'd go right back down and then they'd go off the page again.*

Liver biopsy. The best way to confirm whether or not you have cirrhosis is to undergo a liver biopsy. However, if you have a swollen, fluid-filled belly because of ascites or a tendency to bleed easily because your liver is not producing blood-clotting factors as it should, it can be unsafe for you to have the most common type of liver biopsy: that is, with a needle through the skin (percutaneously). Thus, before your doctor does this procedure, he or she will check whether or not you are at risk for undue bleeding by performing even more blood tests that include prothrombin time (PT), partial thromboplastin time (PTT), platelet count, and sometimes a special test called bleeding time.

If the results of these blood tests show that you are not at risk for bleeding complications, your doctor may recommend that you undergo a liver biopsy and refer you to a specialist. Most often, this type of procedure is done on an outpatient basis by a gastroenterologist or a hepatologist, as it was for Jack. If the results of your blood tests indicate that you *are* at risk for bleeding, your physician may suggest that you undergo one of two other types of liver biopsies: a transvenous or a surgical biopsy. Chapter 2 provides more information about all three types of liver biopsies and how you can prepare for them.

Radiologic studies. Another option, if your risk of bleeding from a liver biopsy is high, is to do a radiologic study instead. For this type of test, your physician may send you to the radiology department of your hospital or clinic for an ultrasound, computed axial tomographic (CAT, or simply CT) scan, or magnetic resonance imaging (MRI) test. Chapter 2 explains how these tests work and what you can expect if you need to have them done.

> By the time I saw a liver specialist, my cirrhosis already was in an advanced stage. After the blood tests, they started with the ultrasounds and the CAT scans, and they saw my enlarged spleen. A biopsy wasn't necessary. It was just so obvious. My liver was scarred and shrinking. It's a progressive disease, and it had started to progress rather rapidly with me.

Sometimes gastroenterologists and hepatologists can make a clinical diagnosis of cirrhosis by virtue of telltale signs on these radiologic studies. For example, if a CAT scan of your abdomen shows a small, shrunken, bumpy (nodular), distorted liver, together with an enlarged spleen, fluid in the abdomen (ascites), and prominent veins around your liver and spleen, you very likely have cirrhosis of the liver.

You may wonder why doctors go to the trouble of performing a liver biopsy if they sometimes can identify cirrhosis with a simple CAT scan. Here it's important to point out that with cirrhosis—as with all liver diseases—a liver biopsy provides the most complete, explicit information about what is happening to your liver on a cellular level. It's the very best diagnostic tool that liver specialists have, so unless you are at risk for bleeding or you have ascites, your physician probably will recommend that you undergo this simple procedure.

HOW SEVERE IS YOUR CIRRHOSIS?

If the results from your biopsy or radiologic tests show that you definitely have cirrhosis, your next question may be, How bad is my liver disease? This is a very good question, because not all cirrhotics are created equal! Hepatologists frequently use the Childs-Pugh classification system to rank the severity of a patient's cirrhosis. This system is based on the results of tests that measure a protein called albumin and a bile pigment called bilirubin in your blood, as well as on prothrombin time, which relates to your blood's ability to clot. A score also is assigned for two possible complications of your liver disease: the presence of fluid in your abdomen (ascites) and mental confusion, which is the hallmark of hepatic encephalopathy, a neurological syndrome that sometimes occurs when the scarred liver can no longer rid the body of certain toxins.

CHILDS CLASS A DISEASE

If your gastroenterologist or hepatologist tells you that you have "Childs class A" disease, you are fortunate enough to have the mildest form of cirrhosis, and you may do well for many years. Major complications (which I'll tell you about later on in this chapter) are unlikely to happen over the next few years, and if need be, you can undergo surgery with general anesthesia without major risks.

CHILDS CLASS B AND C DISEASE

If you have Childs class B or C disease, your cirrhosis has caused considerable damage to your liver, and you have a poorer prognosis than people with Childs class A disease. With such advanced disease, you'll need to be on the lookout for possible complications, and you should be aware that your risks from anesthesia and major surgical procedures are high.

WHAT CAUSED YOUR CIRRHOSIS?

No matter how severe your liver scarring is, your doctor should attempt to find out what caused it, because therapies for these underlying conditions can vary greatly. Let's talk now about the different causes of cirrhosis and their corresponding treatments. I'll begin with the most common causes of this liver disease—alcoholism and certain kinds of hepatitis.

ALCOHOLISM

Alcoholism is responsible for 75 to 80 percent of cases of cirrhosis worldwide. If your cirrhosis was caused by heavy drinking, no medicine you can take will reverse the scarring in your liver. Instead, your primary therapeutic option will require a tremendously difficult personal challenge: you must give up alcohol completely. If you don't, you risk further damage to your liver that eventually could lead to liver failure.

As I said in chapter 8, cirrhosis that is attributable to heavy drinking is one stage in a broader disease process called alcoholic liver disease. Another thing that could happen if you continue to drink alcohol is that your illness could progress to the next stage of this disease: liver cancer. Both liver failure due to alcoholic cirrhosis and liver cancer are expressions of end-stage disease that may require you to have an operation (such as a liver transplant, which is described in detail in chapter 13).

Therefore, if your cirrhosis was caused by alcohol, I recommend that you do everything that you can to stop drinking for good. The support of family and friends, groups such as Alcoholics Anonymous, and private counseling with a licensed social worker or psychotherapist all can be helpful in conquering this major challenge in your life. In chapter 8, you'll find more information about the resources that are available to help you overcome this addiction.

Hepatitis

If you have cirrhosis, it's a good idea to stop drinking alcohol even if alcoholism did not cause your liver disease. Alcohol can act as an accelerator of this disease process, especially in people with hepatitis, or inflammation of the liver.

Different kinds of chronic (long-term) hepatitis can lead to cirrhosis; these include viral hepatitis B, C, and D, autoimmune hepatitis, and alcoholic hepatitis. Some types of viral hepatitis (for example, acute viral hepatitis A and E infections) never lead to long-term liver inflammation or cirrhosis.

Viral hepatitis. As I explained in chapters 3 through 6, hepatitis B and hepatitis C are blood-borne viruses that can be acquired in a number of ways, including intimate sexual contact, use of intravenous drugs, and accidental needle sticks with contaminated syringes. Chronic hepatitis B infection can progress to cirrhosis, although it's not clear how often this occurs in parts of the world where the virus is not prevalent, or endemic. In areas where the virus is endemic (for example, in Southeast Asia and sub-Saharan Africa), current estimates suggest that 10 to 20 percent of patients with chronic HBV will develop cirrhosis. An estimated 25 percent of people with chronic hepatitis C infection go on to develop cirrhosis, typically over many years. Lastly, chronic hepatitis D (delta) infection, which often is linked to hepatitis B infection, carries with it a high (75 percent) risk of developing cirrhosis.

The various types of hepatitis call for different therapeutic measures. If you have chronic hepatitis B infection, for instance, your treatment may consist of the drugs interferon or lamivudine, whereas if you have chronic hepatitis C, your doctor may prescribe a combination of interferon and ribavirin. At present there is no known effective treatment for the hepatitis D viral infection.

Even if you are tested for the hepatitis A and B viruses and your doctor determines that you do *not* have either of these viral infections, you still may need to be vaccinated against them if you have cirrhosis or any other form of liver disease. That's because if you were to acquire one of these infections in addition to your already-existing liver disease, you could become quite ill. We currently have very effective vaccines to prevent hepatitis A and B infection, and the Centers for Disease Control (CDC) Advisory Committee on Vaccination Practices has recommended that all people with chronic liver disease receive them. We hope to have a vaccine for protection against hepatitis C in the near future (see chapter 6).

NONVIRAL HEPATITIS. Liver scarring also may be caused by nonviral diseases such as autoimmune hepatitis and alcoholic hepatitis. You'll find more details about autoimmune hepatitis in chapter 7 and about alcoholic hepatitis, which is one stage of alcoholic liver disease, in chapter 8. For autoimmune hepatitis, corticosteroids such as prednisone can have dramatic and magical effects. Note that for chronic *viral* hepatitis (*not* autoimmune hepatitis), corticosteroids can have detrimental effects, actually worsening your liver disease; this is another reason why it is important for your doctor to determine exactly what is causing your cirrhosis. For alcoholic hepatitis, you will need to stop drinking alcohol completely and perhaps take nutritional supplements and corticosteroids.

GENETIC HEMOCHROMATOSIS

Another cause of cirrhosis is an "iron overload" disorder called hemochromatosis. In this inherited disease, which affects more men than women, excessive amounts of iron are absorbed from the gastrointestinal tract and deposited in organs and tissues such as the liver, pancreas, joints, and heart. Over the years this accumulation can cause cirrhosis, diabetes, arthritis, and heart failure. To get rid of this extra iron, blood is drawn, often on a weekly basis, in a procedure known as phlebotomy. This treatment, which may be repeated for many weeks, months, or even a few years, is described in more detail in chapter 11.

Unfortunately, as many as 25 percent of patients with cirrhosis due to genetic hemochromatosis will develop liver cancer. It's thus critical, if you have this disorder, to see a specialist for continued careful monitoring and treatment.

WILSON'S DISEASE

Another genetic disorder that can lead to cirrhosis—Wilson's disease—is 100 times less common than hemochromatosis. In this condition, copper is not metabolized normally in the body. Consequently, this trace metal is deposited in the eyes, brain, and liver, where it can lead to cirrhosis. If you have Wilson's disease, your doctor probably will prescribe a drug called penicillamine to chelate, or remove, this excess copper. This treatment has to be continued for life, but it is lifesaving! Fortunately, the risk of liver cancer in patients with cirrhosis of the liver due to Wilson's disease is extremely low.

ALPHA$_1$ANTITRYPSIN DEFICIENCY

Another inherited disorder, alpha$_1$antitrypsin deficiency, occurs when the liver doesn't produce enough of a certain plasma protein. This rare protein deficiency may cause lung diseases such as emphysema even in individuals who may not smoke, and it also can lead to cirrhosis. There is no specific treatment for this disorder, but perhaps novel gene therapies will become available in the near future.

PRIMARY BILIARY CIRRHOSIS

Primary biliary cirrhosis (PBC), which I'll discuss at length in the next chapter, is a disorder characterized by destruction of the bile ducts within the liver. Cirrhosis is a somewhat misleading name for this disease; although PBC can lead to cirrhosis, many people when first diagnosed with PBC do *not* have cirrhosis. PBC is not caused by viral infections or alcohol, but instead may be linked to a problem with the body's autoimmune system. It is more common in women than in men.

PBC may cause itching, fatigue, and increased skin pigmentation that can create the appearance of a "healthy tan" even in the dead of winter. About 25 percent of people with this disease also develop significant bone loss (osteoporosis). There is no surefire cure for PBC, but drugs such as ursodeoxycholic acid (ursodiol or Actigall) and colchicine may be helpful in delaying its course. Scientists also are investigating the use of low doses of a drug called methotrexate for people with this disorder.

PRIMARY SCLEROSING CHOLANGITIS

Another disease that affects the bile ducts is primary sclerosing cholangitis (PSC). This disease, which is more common in men than women, is characterized by chronic, progressive narrowing (stricture) and destruction of both the bile ducts within the liver and those that come out of the liver and enter the intestine. The narrowing of these bile ducts causes bile to build up in the liver, and this buildup can lead to scarring, or cirrhosis. If you have PSC, you may suffer from a related disorder called inflammatory bowel disease (also called chronic ulcerative colitis or Crohn's disease).

There is no specific cure for PSC, but we can treat the expressions of this disease. For example, blocked bile flow in the liver can lead to infection, which can be managed with antibiotics. Also, the narrowed bile ducts can be dilated or opened up with cylindrical devices called stents, and sometimes bile can be drained from the liver via a surgical bypass of the obstructed bile ducts. For severe cases, liver transplantation may be necessary.

NONALCOHOLIC STEATOHEPATITIS

Alcoholic hepatitis, as I said earlier, is a liver inflammation caused by long-term consumption of alcohol. If you have this condition and you continue to drink heavily, your illness may progress to the next stage of alcoholic liver disease, which is cirrhosis.

When he is examining a piece of liver tissue (from a biopsy specimen) under the microscope, it can be impossible for a pathologist or hepatologist to tell the difference between the features of alcoholic hepatitis and another condition that has nothing to do with alcohol consumption—nonalcoholic steatohepatitis (NASH). Under the microscope, the cell damage related to these two conditions looks exactly the same: there are extra fat deposits, particular structures known as Mallory's hyaline (previously known as alcoholic hyaline) bodies, and infiltration of the liver cells with infection-fighting white blood cells.

If the clinical picture of these two diseases is the same, how can doctors tell which one you have? The diagnosis depends entirely on whether or not you have consumed enough alcohol to cause liver injury.

Recently I saw a forty-two-year-old diabetic woman named Gina who was referred to me by her internist. When he examined her, he found that she was overweight and that both her liver and spleen were enlarged. Subsequent blood tests showed that she had abnormal liver function tests, or LFTs. He suspected that she might have cirrhosis, and he referred her to me for consultation and consideration of a liver biopsy.

When I performed the biopsy, I discovered that Gina did in fact have cirrhosis. I then met with her to discuss the biopsy results, and I asked about her alcohol consumption. Like Jack, my other patient, she was very surprised at the diagnosis, saying, "But Dr. Chopra, I only drink one or two times a year and only on special occasions. How could I have cirrhosis?" She then described her embarrassment when she told one of her friends recently that her internist had suggested that she might have cirrhosis. The friend had looked at her in a peculiar way, as if she was wondering whether Gina was a closet alcoholic.

I explained to Gina that not all cases of cirrhosis are related to alcohol. I had previously asked her in detail about her history and even spoke with some of her family members, who confirmed that she was not a drinker. She turned out to have NASH.

Like Gina, many people with NASH are overweight women between the ages of forty and sixty years. Often, but not invariably, they also have diabetes mellitus (sometimes called "sugar diabetes"). They have either no symptoms or vague abdominal discomfort and may discover that they have NASH only if they go to see a doctor for an unrelated medical problem.

NASH carries with it a 10 to 20 percent chance of progressing to cirrhosis. There is no proven therapy for this disorder, although I recommend weight loss for overweight patients. Ursodeoxycholic acid, the drug given to patients with PBC, may be helpful. I also recommend 800 international units of vitamin E daily. Phlebotomy (blood letting) may be helpful.

BILIARY ATRESIA AND GLYCOGEN STORAGE DISORDERS

Two other causes of cirrhosis—biliary atresia and glycogen storage disorders—occur only in children. These young patients should be seen by a pediatric gastroenterologist or hepatologist who has expertise in handling such conditions.

We don't know what causes biliary atresia, a congenital disorder that sometimes occurs in children, some of whom have Down syndrome. In children with this liver disorder, the bile ducts both inside and outside the liver are absent or not fully developed. As with the other bile duct disorders that I described earlier, narrowing of these tiny channels can lead to unremitting blockage of the bile that normally should flow out of the liver with ease; this buildup can lead to jaundice and eventually to the development of scar tissue that characterizes cirrhosis.

Treatment for biliary atresia often involves an operation called hepatic portoenterostomy, or the "Kasai operation," named after the Japanese surgeon who invented it. In this procedure, a loop of bowel is used to create a connection from the bile ducts within the liver to the intestine. This operation can provide the child with relief for a number of years, buying time that will allow him to grow sufficiently so that a liver transplant eventually can be done with an increased chance of success.

Glycogen storage disorders are also inherited conditions that can cause cirrhosis. In these disorders, the body is unable to export glycogen from its storage place in the liver to other places where it is needed. A child with a glycogen storage disorder may have a massively enlarged liver and spleen, as well as a low blood glucose level. He or she may fail to grow and may be at risk for the development of benign tumors called hepatic adenomas. In rare instances, these tumors can degenerate and turn into liver cancer (see pages 221–23). The treatment of glycogen storage disorders generally involves liver transplantation, usually with good success.

LESS COMMON CAUSES OF CIRRHOSIS

As I have mentioned, most cases of cirrhosis can be attributed to alcoholism, certain types of hepatitis, and inherited disorders such as genetic hemochromatosis, Wilson's disease, and alpha$_1$antitrypsin deficiency, as well as problems involving the biliary ducts.

Less common conditions, including cardiac cirrhosis and infection with a parasite called *Schistosomatium,* also can lead to cirrhosis. In patients with cardiac cirrhosis, a form of chronic, congestive heart failure leads to a backup of blood flow within the liver. With the passage of time, this liver congestion can cause scarring. With schistosomiasis, the eggs of the *Schistosomatium* parasite lodge in the liver and incite inflammation and the development of scar tissue.

If at first your doctor finds no clear-cut explanation for your cirrhosis, he or she should try to address all of these possible causes before coming to the conclusion that your liver disease is "cryptogenic" (which means he or she is stumped and doesn't know what's causing it). Sometimes drugs such as diuretics or medications for high blood pressure, or vitamin A in excessive amounts, also may lead to cirrhosis if taken over a long period. Thus you can help your physician in this diagnostic process by telling him about *all* medications that you are taking, even if you have been taking them in such low doses or for such a long time that they no longer seem worth mentioning.

Finally, if you have had any usual exposure to potentially toxic chemicals, either at home or at work, you should let your doctor know. These causes of cirrhosis, though extremely rare, are worth pursuing.

A FINAL NOTE ON THE CAUSE OF YOUR CIRRHOSIS

Because so many different conditions can lead to liver scarring, and there are so many different treatments for these underlying disorders, you can see why accurately determining the cause of your cirrhosis is so crucial. Careful testing with a qualified gastrointestinal or liver specialist is very important.

In the process of your diagnostic workup, what if your doctor finds that you have hepatitis C virus infection, or, when you tell him about your medical history, it becomes clear that you drink more alcohol than you should? Should you and your physician jump to the conclusion that your cirrhosis was caused by your HCV infection or by alcoholism? Not necessarily.

Given the number of disparate factors that can be responsible for cirrhosis, it's possible that you may have, for example, a mild case of hepatitis C that is not causing your cirrhosis, but a coexisting case of an iron overload disorder (hemochromatosis) that is. Since treatments for these two conditions are entirely different, treatment for only one of them would be less than desirable.

It thus can be useful to be informed about the various causes of cirrhosis (see the box on page 163), and you should ask your doctor if you

---

Causes of Cirrhosis

1. Alcoholism
2. Chronic hepatitis B virus (HBV) infection, with or without chronic hepatitis D virus (HDV) infection
3. Chronic hepatitis C virus (HCV) infection
4. Nonalcoholic steatohepatitis (NASH)
5. Genetic hemochromatosis
6. Primary biliary cirrhosis
7. Autoimmune hepatitis
8. Wilson's disease
9. Alpha$_1$antitrypsin deficiency
10. Primary sclerosing cholangitis
11. Biliary atresia
12. Glycogen storage disorders
13. Cardiac cirrhosis
14. Prolonged exposure to environmental toxins
15. Severe reaction to certain drugs
16. Schistosomiasis (parasitic infection)

Note: Hepatitis A and E do *not* lead to cirrhosis.

---

are concerned that you may have more than one risk factor for this type of liver disease. He may need to perform a comprehensive battery of blood tests. Your liver biopsy also may reveal characteristic or even diagnostic features of a particular liver disorder.

FAMILY RAMIFICATIONS

In addition to the significant prognostic and therapeutic consequences that the cause of your cirrhosis will have for you, there also may be important ramifications for your family. If you have a chronic infection with the hepatitis B or hepatitis C virus, for instance, your family members should be tested to see if they are infected. If so, they may need to see a gastroenterologist or hepatologist. Also, if you have HBV infection, your family members should be screened, and if they do *not* have the virus or protective antibodies (immunity), they still may need to be vaccinated against it (there is no available vaccine to prevent HCV infection).

Finally, if the cause of your cirrhosis is an inherited disorder like hemochromatosis or Wilson's disease, the condition could have been passed on genetically to your children, and they should be screened for the disease. Likewise, your siblings may be affected, and they should be screened, too.

COMPLICATIONS OF CIRRHOSIS

You now know that the treatment of your cirrhosis is linked to identifying the cause of the cirrhosis and, if the cause is treatable, taking the appropriate remedy. The management of your cirrhosis also may involve treating the complications of this disorder.

The complications of cirrhosis can be dramatic, frightening, or alarming to patients and family members, and even potentially life-threatening. They range from fluid accumulation within the abdomen to infection, bleeding, mental confusion, kidney failure, and even liver cancer. Each of these complications and the treatments for them are described below.

ASCITES

The word *ascites* is derived from the Greek word *askos,* which means "bag." This term refers to a buildup of fluid in the abdomen. Ascites may cause you to gain weight and develop a markedly distended belly, so that you may look "pregnant."

Generally, I suspect that one of the "five Fs" is responsible when one of my patients has generalized abdominal distention: fat, feces, fluid, flatus (gas), or fetus! With ascites, the *F* is fluid that comes both from the surface of the liver and from the intestines. The amount of fluid that accumulates in the abdomen is higher than the amount of fluid that the body's lymphatic system can remove. The mechanism of ascites formation is complex, and there are a variety of causes; these include congestive heart failure and malignancy, as well as liver disease. If your ascites is caused by cirrhosis, you probably will have obvious abdominal swelling. Your doctor can confirm the diagnosis of ascites by performing an ultrasound or abdominal CT scan, or by removal of the fluid using a sterile technique called paracentesis.

Sometimes cirrhosis causes portal hypertension (or increased pressure in the liver's system of portal veins, which transport blood from the stomach, spleen, and intestines to the liver. When this increased pressure occurs, fluid can accumulate in the abdominal cavity. The kidneys also will retain sodium and water, leading to further aggravation of this condition. Other complications of ascites include breathing problems (caused by the upward pressure of the enlarged abdomen) and infection of the ascitic fluid, a condition called spontaneous bacterial peritonitis (SBP).

This infection may have led to the demise of the great composer Beethoven. In a classic article about SBP, Dr. Harold Conn, an eminent hepatologist at Yale, recounts that Beethoven suffered from ascites. Toward the end of his life, he became ill and had jaundice, chills, fever, abdominal pain, and a tremendous thirst. In order to relieve the great amount of fluid that had accumulated in Beethoven's abdomen, his surgeon advocated puncture, or paracentesis, "to preclude the danger of sudden bursting." Almost twenty-five pounds of liquid were removed, and the afterflow was estimated to have been five times that. When Beethoven saw the stream of fluid that was released, he "cried out happily that the operation made him think of Moses, who struck the rock with his staff and made the water gush forth." He experienced almost immediate relief.

However, inflammation set in, and Beethoven's doctors noted that he had signs of gangrene. They tried to drain his ascitic fluid three more times, but the fluid soon reaccumulated. As with paracentesis today, these procedures had only a palliative effect; in other words, they alleviated some discomfort but did not cure the underlying liver disease that caused the ascites. Records indicate that Beethoven received the last rites on March 24, 1827. He died peacefully two days later at the age of fifty-seven.

Two doctors at the Pathology Museum of the Vienna Anatomical Institute performed an autopsy on Beethoven's body and found that it was wasted and covered with bruises. His liver was shrunk to half volume, leathery, and had surface bumps, or nodules. His spleen was twice the normal size, and his pancreas was enlarged and hardened. The autopsy thus confirmed that Beethoven, though a legendary giant in the eyes of many, nevertheless lacked the regenerative powers that had saved the mythological hero Prometheus.

If your cirrhosis has caused ascites, there are many more treatment options available to you than there were to Beethoven. Today ascites can be treated in the following ways:

- By restricting salt in your diet (to 2,000 mg per day).
- With drugs called diuretics, which can help your body to get rid of excess fluid by increasing your output of urine. Two commonly pre-scribed diuretics are spironolactone (Aldactone) and furosemide (Lasix).
- With repeated draining of your ascitic fluid by large-volume para-centesis (as was performed years ago for Beethoven). During this procedure, your doctor will insert a needle into your abdomen, and up to several liters of ascitic fluid will be removed. Just as with Beethoven, this procedure will not treat the underlying condition, and the fluid will simply build up again. Paracentesis also has minor associated risks and can be expensive.
- With a LeVeen (or Denver) shunt, which transfers fluid through a tube that is tunneled underneath the skin from the peritoneal cav-ity (abdomen) to the heart. This surgical procedure has many related complications, and I seldom recommend it.
- With placement of a device called a transvenous intrahepatic por-tosystemic shunt or stent (TIPS) into the liver. This procedure is per-formed only for patients with ascites that does not improve with other forms of treatment. It requires the expertise of radiologists with special training and is best performed in centers where there is considerable experience.

    This is how it works: A radiologist inserts a small catheter into a vein in your neck. This catheter is then directed to the liver, where a stent is placed between the portal and hepatic veins. Once in place, this device facilitates blood flow and thus lowers the ele-vated pressure in your liver's system of portal veins.

    Before undergoing a TIPS procedure, you and your family should discuss its associated risks and complications with a hepa-tologist or gastroenterologist. One major risk of the procedure is bleeding, and a major complication is the worsening or development of a syndrome called hepatic encephalopathy (see pages 170–71). Just as with paracentesis, shunts and stents will not cure the cirrhosis that caused your ascites. Although they often relieve the buildup of fluid, the fluid may reaccumulate quickly.

- By liver transplantation, if you are an acceptable candidate (see chapter 13).

VARICEAL BLEEDING

Unlike the healthy liver of Prometheus, when a cirrhotic liver tries to regenerate itself, there can be dire consequences. Part of the regenerative process of cirrhosis involves the formation of nodules, or islands of liver tissue totally encapsulated by scar tissue. The nodules and scar tissue can interfere with the flow of blood to the liver. Blood is thus diverted away from the liver, and prominent collateral blood vessels are opened up.

If you have cirrhosis, you may develop these prominent veins, or varices, in your esophagus. If these engorged veins rupture, you may vomit blood or pass blood through the rectum. Variceal bleeding occurs in 25 to 40 percent of people who have cirrhosis. This is a true medical emergency that requires immediate attention.

> *I knew something was wrong, but I didn't know how wrong. It's just a feeling that you have. And all of a sudden I was throwing up all this blood. My husband rushed me to the emergency room, where they used a fairly new procedure to make the bleeding stop. They put rubber bands through a tube that was inserted through my mouth and went down into my esophagus. Then they tightened the rubber bands around the varices to stop the bleeding.*

I like to think of management of variceal bleeding in three scenarios. First: you may have cirrhosis but have never bled from varices. If this is the case, your doctor will need to determine if you do in fact have varices, and if so, what your risk of bleeding is. Second: you already may be experiencing acute bleeding. Third: your acute bleeding episode has been controlled. What can be done to prevent rebleeding in the future?

Let's address the first scenario. Once the diagnosis of cirrhosis has been established, doctors can determine your risk of variceal bleeding by using the Childs-Pugh classification system combined with findings from a procedure called an endoscopy. This procedure can be performed safely in an outpatient setting. You will not be allowed to eat for eight hours before an endoscopy. When you get to the endoscopy suite, you will be given a mild intravenous sedative such as midazolam (Versed) or fentanyl, or both. The endoscopist (most commonly a gastroenterologist or hepatologist) will insert a fiber-optic rubber tube through your mouth into your esophagus, and will determine by looking at an attached video screen whether or not you have esophageal varices. If so, he or she will assess these engorged veins for size and features such as "cherry red" spots and streaks or ridges called red wale markings.

Studies have demonstrated that people with Child's class A cirrhosis, small varices, and lack of certain specific endoscopic features such as red wale markings will have a less than 10 percent risk of bleeding from these varices over the next two-year period. In contrast, if you have more advanced disease and prominent varices, your risk of bleeding is much higher. People with Childs class C cirrhosis, large varices, and prominent red wale markings have a much higher risk (close to 70 percent) of bleeding over the following two years.

If you have prominent varices, your doctor may prescribe drugs called beta blockers to decrease your risk of bleeding. One such medication, which also is used to treat high blood pressure, is propranolol (Inderal).

The second scenario is that you already are experiencing acute bleeding. In this case, you must be treated in an intensive care unit (ICU), where you probably will be given a medication called somatostatin. In addition, you may need to receive blood transfusions and fresh frozen plasma. A technique called endoscopic sclerotherapy may be done to stop the bleeding. In this procedure, the specialist will insert an endoscope into your esophagus, and then she will inject a chemical into the bleeding varices to obliterate them. This procedure may have to be done several times.

In a new procedure that appears to be superior to sclerotherapy—endoscopic band ligation—rubber bands are attached to the end of the endoscope and are used to tie off the bleeding varices.

Sclerotherapy and endoscopic band ligation are effective in arresting acute variceal bleeding in most people. If your bleeding continues despite these efforts, a method known as TIPS (transvenous intrahepatic portosystemic shunt) can be used to stop the bleeding (this method also is used for the management of ascites; see page 166–67).

Balloon tamponade is another technique that can be used if you are still bleeding a great deal in spite of some of the above-mentioned procedures or while you are being transferred from a small community hospital to a major medical center. In this procedure, a tube with esophageal and gastric balloons will be inserted into your stomach, and the balloons will then be inflated to apply pressure (tamponade) to the ruptured varices.

Once your variceal bleeding has been brought under control, there are several ways to prevent rebleeding. They include:

- Drugs called beta blockers.
- Endoscopic band ligation (to tie off the varices that may rebleed).
- Transvenous intrahepatic portosystemic shunt (TIPS). Your hepatologist or gastroenterologist may recommend this procedure as a very effective "bridge" to stabilize you prior to a liver transplant.
- Liver transplantation (see chapter 13).

BLEEDING TENDENCY

Your liver has several important functions, including the production of factors that are essential for your blood to clot. With cirrhosis, your liver may not produce these clotting factors adequately, so you may develop nosebleeds, bleeding gums, and excessive internal bleeding. Like Beethoven, you also may bruise easily.

If you have a significant blood-clotting impairment, it's imperative that you not engage in contact sports or pursue hobbies such as bungee jumping! You should also scrupulously avoid aspirin and scores of other "blood-thinning" drugs called nonsteroidal anti-inflammatory agents (NSAIDS). These drugs include common agents such as ibuprofen (Motrin, Advil), naproxyn sodium (Aleve), and ketoprofen (Orudis KT and Actron).

HEPATIC ENCEPHALOPATHY

Another important function of your liver is to serve as a "detoxification plant" that clears your body of a number of noxious substances that accumulate in the simple process of digestion of foods. One important toxin is ammonia. If you have cirrhosis, your liver may not be able to perform this critical task, so ammonia can build up in your body. This buildup can eventually affect your central nervous system and cause a condition known as hepatic encephalopathy. Symptoms of this syndrome range from mild confusion and personality changes to frank coma. Some patients also experience restlessness, euphoria, and altered sleep rhythms.

> *A year after my wife was hospitalized with a variceal bleed, we were in New York to see her brother, and she came down with her first noticeable case of encephalopathy. It was the night after Christmas, and we had just returned from having dinner out. She became disoriented and confused. I found her wandering around outside of the apartment, in the hallway, looking for the bathroom. I called the medical center, and they said to give her lactulose. I gave it to her immediately and took her to the emergency room. They told me not to stop to fill out insurance forms at the front desk of the hospital, because she was at risk for going into hepatic coma.*

If your cirrhosis causes hepatic encephalopathy, your liver specialist can diagnose this condition based on:

- The presence of liver disease (according to your physical examination findings, blood tests, and possibly a liver biopsy)
- Symptoms of confusion and restlessness
- Tremors and muscle contractions
- A low body temperature (hypothermia); abnormally prolonged, rapid, and deep breathing (hyperventilation); and a peculiar musty, fruity, and pungent breath odor

- High levels of ammonia in your blood*
- Abnormal findings on an electroencephalogram (EEG)*
- Your favorable response to appropriate treatment such as lactulose, a sugary syrup

Various factors can trigger and worsen hepatic encephalopathy. They include gastrointestinal bleeding; the use of sedatives and tranquilizers; constipation; accumulation in the blood of toxins that ordinarily are eliminated by the kidneys (this occurs in a condition called uremia); and infection. Consumption of a high-protein meal also may be to blame for the mental confusion that marks this syndrome. To remind my patients and their families about this connection, I sometimes quote the great bard William Shakespeare, who wrote, "I am a great eater of beef, and I believe that does harm to my wit" (*Twelfth Night* I.iii.92).

To treat your hepatic encephalopathy, your doctor may need to admit you to the hospital. She will try to identify and correct the factors that triggered this condition (for example, by reducing your protein consumption, treating an infection, stopping your gastrointestinal bleeding, or stopping the offending sedative or tranquilizer). Many people also respond favorably to treatment with lactulose.

> *There's a lot of confusion about lactulose—no pun intended. I've met other patients who don't realize that the reason they're taking lactulose is to prevent confusion. If you feel that your mind's racing and you can't really concentrate, talk to your doctor, because you may need to increase your lactulose.*

Finally, sometimes we prescribe an antibiotic called neomycin for patients with hepatic encephalopathy, although we do so with great care, because long-term use of this drug may cause deafness and kidney problems.

---

*These findings are not necessary to make the diagnosis in most people.

ANEMIA

If you have cirrhosis of the liver, you also may have anemia, or a deficiency of red blood cells, because your enlarged spleen may trap these cells as they attempt to circulate through it. Significant blood loss from hemorrhaging varices can cause this problem, too.

If there is increased pressure in the portal veins, which carry blood from the stomach and spleen to the liver, the lining of the stomach may become congested, and more subtle bleeding may occur. This congestion is sometimes referred to as portal hypertensive gastropathy or congestive gastropathy. For anemia due to bleeding varices or congestive gastropathy, blood transfusions may be required to replace the red blood cells that have been lost.

The alcohol that may cause cirrhosis can also lead to anemia, because alcoholics who are malnourished may not consume enough of a vitamin called folic acid. Alcohol also can suppress the bone marrow, the "factory" that produces these cells. With abstinence from alcohol, red-blood-cell levels can improve.

HEPATORENAL SYNDROME

Another complication of cirrhosis, hepatorenal syndrome, is a perplexing, enigmatic, and unexplained problem involving kidney failure in people with very severe end-stage cirrhosis of the liver, but no other known cause of renal failure. The kidneys themselves are inherently normal. In fact, if a patient with hepatorenal syndrome dies, his kidneys can be transplanted into a patient with kidney failure, and they will work! Also, if a patient with hepatorenal syndrome receives a liver transplant, his kidneys will start working again.

There is no effective treatment for this condition, and without liver transplantation, the prognosis for people who have it is poor. However, researchers are looking into potential therapies.

HEPATOPULMONARY SYNDROME

Rarely, patients with cirrhosis also have an unusual and somewhat complex disorder called hepatopulmonary syndrome. If you have this syndrome, you may experience shortness of breath when sitting up and gain relief only when lying down.

To diagnose hepatopulmonary syndrome, your physician may have you undergo a special blood test. In this procedure, a sterile needle will be inserted into one of the superficial arteries in your arm. The blood that is drawn will be sent to the laboratory for analysis of your blood oxygen levels, as well as your blood's pH, which reflects the acid-base balance of your body. You may also need to have a simple and painless imaging test called a contrast echocardiogram. In this test, ultrasound waves are sent through your chest wall and "echo" back from the inside of your heart to provide a picture of the motion of your heart and its surrounding tissues.

Treatment of hepatopulmonary syndrome is evolving and includes oxygen supplementation and specialized shunt procedures such as TIPS. A preliminary pilot study published in 1998 also suggests that garlic may improve symptoms and oxygen levels in people with hepatopulmonary syndrome. What an intriguing finding! Further investigation clearly is warranted.

LIVER CANCER

Liver cancer, which is also called primary liver cancer, primary hepatocellular carcinoma, and hepatoma, refers to cancer that arises in the liver, not to cancer that originates in another organ such as the breast, lung, or colon and then metastasizes (spreads) to the liver.

Although most people with primary liver cancer have cirrhosis, the majority of people with cirrhosis will *not* develop liver cancer even ten years after their liver scarring is diagnosed. Your risk of developing liver cancer is greatest if your cirrhosis was caused by a chronic hepatitis B or hepatitis C viral infection or genetic hemochromatosis. In contrast, if you have alcoholic cirrhosis or primary biliary cirrhosis (PBC), you have a low to intermediate risk of developing liver cancer. People with cirrhosis due to Wilson's disease, autoimmune hepatitis, or nonalcoholic steatohepatitis (NASH) rarely develop liver cancer.

Your doctor may want to monitor you for the development of liver cancer by performing a readily available blood test called alpha-fetoprotein (AFP). This test to screen for a "tumor marker" is often done at periodic intervals (two to three times per year). A dedicated liver ultrasound or a CAT scan of the liver also can be done periodically (every six months or so) in the expectation and hope that no tumor will be found. If a tumor is found, however, it may be discovered at an early stage, at which point it can be removed by a surgical procedure called a partial hepatectomy. The treatment of liver cancer is described in further detail in chapter 12.

SUMMARY

Now you know what cirrhosis is, how it is diagnosed, and how its various causes and complications can be managed. If you've been diagnosed with cirrhosis, you may want to take the following list along next time you visit your gastroenterologist or liver specialist to help you remember which key questions to ask:

- What caused my cirrhosis? Should members of my family be concerned about having the same risk factor or factors?
- How severe is my cirrhosis (is it Childs class A, B, or C)?
- Is there a specific treatment available for my disease?
- Should I make any changes in my lifestyle? Do I need to give up alcohol?
- Do I need to receive the HAV or HBV vaccine?
- Do I have esophageal varices? If so, what is my risk of bleeding? Should I be taking any medicine to prevent variceal bleeding?
- Do I have any other complications of cirrhosis such as ascites, hepatic encephalopathy, or liver cancer?
- Should I have periodic screening for liver cancer?

Your doctor should be able to answer these questions, and he or she will be able to find the treatment plan that is exactly right for you. You and your family should feel encouraged to know that dedicated and brilliant scientists in many parts of the world are studying many aspects of cirrhosis and that important breakthroughs will likely occur in the foreseeable future.

10

Primary Biliary Cirrhosis

My husband started to call me "Lady Macbeth" because I was washing the sheets, towels, and my clothes constantly. I was itching all over and I was convinced that I had developed an allergy, so I threw away the soaps and laundry detergents that we'd been using and tried various products for sensitive skin— but nothing seemed to help.

Finally, the itching that had been just annoying at first became quite irritating, so I called my primary care doctor, who I hadn't seen for a number of years, and went to visit her. She did some tests, and I was expecting her to give me a referral to a dermatologist. Instead she gave me a referral to a hepatologist because she said that I may have a liver disease called primary biliary cirrhosis.

She tried to reassure me that I may not have cirrhosis, but rather a disease that potentially could turn into cirrhosis. I'm glad that she made that distinction, because I was so astonished by the diagnosis at first—"Cirrhosis" was the only word that sunk in.

—JENNIFER HURLEY, age forty-two

Primary biliary cirrhosis (PBC) is a chronic (long-lasting) disorder characterized by the gradual, progressive destruction of bile ducts within the liver. Although it eventually can develop into liver scarring (cirrhosis) and lead to liver failure, you shouldn't panic if you've just been diagnosed with PBC; treatments are available to slow down the course of this disease, and some people do well for many years with little or no apparent disease progression.

When I evaluated Jennifer, blood tests and a liver biopsy confirmed that she had PBC. Luckily, her biopsy showed that she did not have cirrhosis. Indeed, many people, like Jennifer, do not have cirrhosis when their PBC is first diagnosed; hence, *primary biliary cirrhosis* is a somewhat misleading term. However, the alternative name—pleomorphic nonsuppurative destructive cholangitis—is quite a mouthful!

ARE YOU AT RISK?

The cause of PBC is not known, but we do know that it's not related to alcohol consumption or to chronic viral hepatitis—two very common causes of cirrhosis. Rather, scientists suspect that PBC may have something to do with an abnormality in the body's regulation of the immune system. That's because PBC often coexists with autoimmune conditions such as hypothyroidism. *Autoimmunity* means that the body is marshaling a defensive response to some of its own cells and tissues; as a result, the normal functions of these cells and tissues may be altered. For example, a misguided immune response may cause inflammation of the thyroid gland, or "autoimmune thyroiditis." An underactive thyroid condition (hypothyroidism) may develop if this gland can no longer produce adequate amounts of thyroid hormone. Researchers also are trying to figure out whether there is a genetic component to PBC, because it's been known to occur in more than one member of a family.

PBC is seen in individuals between the ages of twenty and eighty years, although most people are between forty and sixty years old when their disease is first diagnosed, and roughly 90 percent of people with PBC are women. PBC occurs in all parts of the world, with several thousand cases in the United States.

SYMPTOMS

Like more than half of all people with this condition, you may have no symptoms when your PBC is first diagnosed, even though you may turn out to have signs of advanced disease (such as cirrhosis) when a liver biopsy is done. Even if you don't have any indications of illness at the time of diagnosis, you most likely will develop symptoms within a few years.

The common symptoms of PBC—itching all over the body, fatigue, and "tanned" skin caused by increased pigmentation—relate to long-term blockage of bile flow in the liver (this is called cholestasis). Destruction of the small bile ducts in this important organ can further impair the flow of bile out of the liver and into the intestine. Bile acids, a pigment called bilirubin, and copper are then retained within the liver, where their buildup causes damage.

Let's take a closer look at these and other symptoms of PBC, any of which may develop with the passage of time.

ITCHING

If you have PBC, the following poem may resonate with you:

> *There was a young belle of old Natchez*
> *Whose garments were always in patchez.*
> *When comment arose*
> *On the state of her clothes,*
> *She drawled, When Ah itchez, Ah scratchez!*
> —OGDEN NASH

Do you feel as if you need to scratch constantly? Is your itching interfering with work and sleep? If so, you should visit your doctor, who will be able to tell very easily with a simple blood test if you have a liver disorder.

As recently as a few decades ago, though, these diagnostic blood tests were not performed routinely. If you went to your doctor and said that you were suffering from annoying itching, he might have examined you, found no clues pointing to a liver problem, and sent you to a dermatologist. The dermatologist, in turn, would not have found any skin disorder, and he may have suggested that you see a psychiatrist!

If you have PBC, though, you know that the itching is *not* all in your head. It's a very real malady, although the mechanism that causes it is not perfectly well understood. The itching of PBC, which may be mild or debilitating, is usually worse at bedtime and can interfere with your sleep. Chronic itching and scratching also may cause you to lose skin elasticity and may lead to an increase in skin pigmentation, so that you may appear to have a "healthy tan" that does not fade in the winter months.

Sometimes this itching begins when a patient is pregnant or taking birth control pills. However, if you develop this symptom during pregnancy, you may have a condition that is unrelated to an underlying liver problem, or you may have another liver disorder that has no connection to PBC, such as intrahepatic cholestasis of pregnancy. This more common liver condition is seen worldwide but is most prevalent in Chile, India, and the Scandinavian countries. Unlike PBC, the itching of intrahepatic cholestasis of pregnancy abates dramatically after the birth of the newborn.

In any case, your doctor will be able to determine the cause of your itching by doing appropriate blood tests. Later on in this chapter, I'll tell you about treatment options for this irritating symptom.

FATIGUE

Up to two-thirds of people with PBC experience another common and bona fide symptom of this disorder: fatigue. However, tiredness may be caused by many other health problems such as anemia, stress, thyroid disorders, or depression. One study showed that at any given time, 18 percent of the general population may have fatigue that lasts more than six months. For this reason, patients and doctors sometimes dismiss this symptom or attribute it to some of the above-mentioned conditions.

JAUNDICE

Itching and fatigue often precede another classic symptom of PBC: jaundice, or yellowing of the skin and whites of the eyes. You most likely won't have jaundice when your disease is diagnosed. Rather, this symptom usually signals progression of PBC to an advanced stage.

Just as with itching and weariness, though, having jaundice does not necessarily mean that you have PBC or, if you do, that it is at an advanced stage. Jaundice can occur whenever your liver is not doing a good job of removing a bile pigment called bilirubin from your blood. Thus, in addition to PBC, an elevated bilirubin level may be caused by gallstones, infection, inherited disorders of bilirubin metabolism (such as Gilbert's syndrome), untreated thyroid disease, or drug-induced liver injury.

DIARRHEA AND WEIGHT LOSS

Another potential effect of PBC is an alteration in bile salt concentrations; this change can affect your body's ability to absorb fat. If you develop this malabsorption problem, you may experience diarrhea and weight loss.

SYMPTOMS OF CIRRHOSIS

If you have PBC, you may have any of the common symptoms that I just mentioned, as well as any of the classic symptoms of cirrhosis such as weakness and a tendency to bruise easily. On occasion I see a patient who does not seek medical assistance until her PBC is already in a very advanced stage. By this point she may be experiencing a dramatic and even frightening complication of cirrhosis. One such complication—variceal bleeding—occurs when blood flow to the liver is blocked by scar tissue. When this happens, large blood vessels called varices may become engorged in the esophagus. If these varices burst, the severe bleeding that ensues will require immediate medical attention.

Another complication of advanced liver disease is abdominal distention that occurs when fluid accumulates from the surface of the diseased liver and the intestines (this condition is called ascites; see chapter 9). In some instances this swelling can become so great that the patient looks pregnant.

In severe cases of cirrhosis, the patient's liver may fail to rid his or her body of toxic substances that eventually can affect the brain; the resulting condition, called hepatic encephalopathy, can cause mental confusion, personality changes, and even coma.

SYMPTOMS OF RELATED DISORDERS

In addition to the indications of PBC that I have just described, you may find that you have symptoms of other conditions that sometimes go hand in hand with this disease. Here are the important ones to be aware of:

- **Gallstones** may be accompanied by upper abdominal pain.
- **Osteoporosis,** or bone loss, may cause bone pain.
- **High cholesterol** can manifest itself as cholesterol deposits under the skin surface, so that you may find bumps on your eyelids, palms, soles, elbows, knees, ankles, wrists, or buttocks. Most often these bumps are not painful.
- **Iron deficiency anemia** can lead to weakness and a tendency to become fatigued easily.
- **Autoimmune disorders** such as thyroid dysfunction and "dry gland" syndrome (the latter also is called sicca or Sjögren's syndrome) are the most common autoimmune disorders associated with PBC; a few others such as celiac sprue are relatively uncommon. With hypothyroidism, you may have coarse, dry skin and hair; loss of energy; weight gain; and sensitivity to cold. If you have dry gland syndrome, your eyes and mouth may feel uncomfortably dry, so that it may be difficult to eat foods such as dry crackers. Celiac sprue, a disorder that causes malabsorption of nutrients from the intestine, can cause diarrhea and abdominal distention.
- **CRST syndrome** (pronounced "crest syndrome") and *dermatomyositis* are rheumatic conditions; that is, they involve pain or inflammation in the joints, skin, and sometimes muscles. Patients with CRST can have calcium deposits in the skin, pain in or thickening of the skin of the toes and fingers, and small, red lesions on the skin. Dermatomyositis can cause inflammation and a rash on the face, neck, chest, and arms.

Although you probably won't have any of these related disorders, it's important to be aware of them so that you can tell your doctor if you develop any of these symptoms.

Next let's talk about how doctors diagnose PBC and about the kinds of treatments that are available.

DIAGNOSIS

PHYSICAL EXAMINATION

You may discover that you have PBC if you go to your primary care physician because you are experiencing any of the symptoms that I have just described, or you may have no symptoms, and during a routine physical examination your doctor may suspect that you have a liver disorder because he or she finds that you have an enlarged liver or spleen. Your physician also may notice that you have certain telltale manifestations of chronic liver disease such as jaundice, spiderlike skin lesions (spider nevi), red palms (palmar erythema), and "clubbing" of your fingernails, or he may realize that you have PBC because you have fatty bumps caused by cholesterol deposits in your skin and increased skin pigmentation that is causing you to sport a "healthy suntan."

LABORATORY TESTS

If your physical examination leads your doctor to suspect that you may have PBC, he almost certainly will have your blood drawn to diagnose your disease and to find out how extensive it is. The results of blood tests that are done as part of a routine annual checkup also may call attention to your liver disease. These blood tests usually include the following:

- **Complete blood count (CBC),** to look for a deficiency of red blood cells, or anemia. In the early stages of primary biliary cirrhosis, the CBC should be normal. With more advanced disease, however, some patients can develop anemia as a consequence of either obvious or subtle gastrointestinal blood loss. This loss can occur because of hemorrhaging veins, or varices in the esophagus. Milder bleeding may be caused by congestion in the lining of the stomach due to increased pressure in the portal veins that carry blood from the stomach and spleen to the liver. This condition is called congestive gastropathy. If the spleen is enlarged, it also may be contributing to anemia by taking red blood cells captive as they attempt to pass through it.

- **Prothrombin time (PT),** which relates to your blood's clotting ability. The PT is usually normal in the early stages of PBC. If the PT is elevated, your body may not be absorbing vitamin K correctly, or you may have a liver problem such as PBC.

- **Platelet count,** which may be abnormally low if you have developed cirrhosis (see chapter 9).

- **The liver enzymes alanine aminotransferase (ALT) and aspartate aminotransferase (AST).** These tests of liver function, which measure enzymes that are released by damaged liver cells, may be normal or mildly increased if you have PBC.

- **Alkaline phosphatase,** an enzyme level that is almost always significantly elevated in people with PBC. This high level may be related to blockage of the bile ducts within the liver, and this may be the only abnormal liver function test (LFT) result if your disease is in an early stage.

- **Albumin,** a protein that the liver produces and that is usually present in normal levels in early stages of PBC.

- **Bilirubin,** a bile pigment in your blood that is usually present in normal levels early in the disease but increases as the disease worsens.

- **Antimitochondrial antibody (AMA),** which is a convenient marker for PBC because it is positive in more than 90 percent of people with this condition. The nature of this antibody and the relationship between it and the bile duct injury of PBC are not clear. The presence and amount (titer) of AMA do not relate to the severity or course of PBC, and they do not appear to affect the outcome of treatment with a drug called ursodeoxycholic acid or liver transplantation (I'll discuss these treatment options later in this chapter).

- **Serum immunoglobulin (IgM),** a type of protein that also is elevated in about 90 percent of patients with PBC.
- **Serum cholesterol,** which is elevated in 75 percent of people with PBC, often dramatically and strikingly, sometimes to 400–1000 mg/dl (the normal level is less than 200 mg/dl). Although you and even your doctor may be alarmed to discover that your cholesterol level is this high, you should be assured that most often this elevated cholesterol is composed predominantly of high-density lipoprotein (HDL), which is *protective* against coronary artery disease. I've had patients with marked and persistent elevations in serum cholesterol (greater than 400 or 600 mg/dl) who have not had chest pain (angina) or a heart attack (myocardial infarction). One potential side effect of this high cholesterol, though, is that this substance can leave fatty deposits in the skin (see page 190).
- **Screening for the hepatitis A and B viruses,** which should be done if you are found to have PBC. You may need to be vaccinated against both of these viruses, because if you acquire one of these viral infections on top of your already existing liver condition, you could become very ill.

LIVER BIOPSY

Once your primary care physician suspects that you have a liver disorder, he or she may refer you to a liver specialist (a hepatologist) or a specialist in disorders of the gastrointestinal system (a gastroenterologist) to establish the diagnosis and offer appropriate guidelines for management of your condition.

The next step in the diagnostic process is most often a percutaneous (through-the-skin) needle liver biopsy, which is a means of getting a small sample of your liver tissue so that the diagnosis of PBC can be confirmed and the severity of your disease can be determined. Chapter 2 provides more details about liver biopsies and how you can prepare for this procedure.

A pathologist and your hepatologist or gastroenterologist will examine the liver biopsy specimen under the microscope. Depending on the microscopic, or "histologic," features present, they can assign a stage to your disease. Table 10-1 describes the different stages of PBC.

TABLE 10-1

Stages of Primary Biliary Cirrhosis

Stage	Histologic features
I	Asymmetrical destructive lesions of the bile ducts (also called florid duct lesions). These lesions are characteristic of PBC.
II	Fewer normal bile ducts and more small, abnormal, poorly formed bile ducts than usual.
III	Few if any bile ducts and progressive scarring (fibrosis). These features are characteristic, but not diagnostic, of PBC.
IV	Established cirrhosis, with regenerating nodules surrounding liver cells (see chapter 9). It may be impossible to tell from a liver biopsy whether your cirrhosis was caused by PBC or by some other disease process, although an absence of bile ducts in the scarred areas of your liver may suggest PBC.

How Bad Is Your PBC?

With your liver biopsy results in hand, your liver specialist will be able to tell you how severe your disease is and in general what you can expect in terms of a prognosis. As I said earlier, some patients with mild PBC can do well for many years with only slow or little disease progression. If your disease is advanced, however, you may have liver scarring (cirrhosis) that could lead to some serious and even life-threatening complications such as swollen veins (varices) in your esophagus. If you have PBC, it's a good idea to have a procedure called upper endoscopy periodically to look for these varices. This procedure is described in detail in chapter 9. If any varices are found, your doctor may prescribe drugs called beta blockers to prevent them from bleeding.

Like many of my patients, you may have heard that liver cancer can occur with cirrhosis, and you may be alarmed about the possibility of developing this complication. I would assure you that generally the risk of liver cancer associated with PBC is low (less than 10 percent), and good screening methods are available to detect this type of cancer in its early stages, so that if a tumor is found it can be removed successfully. Chapter 12 describes the diagnosis and treatment of primary cancer of the liver in more detail.

TREATMENT

DRUG THERAPY

There is no proven cure for PBC, but if your disease is diagnosed in its early stages, drugs such as ursodeoxycholic acid, colchicine, and perhaps methotrexate may be beneficial. Ursodeoxycholic acid (UDCA; also called Actigall or ursodiol) slows the progression of PBC and may lengthen the time before a patient with PBC may need to undergo a liver transplant. This medication is extremely well tolerated and often relieves the itching associated with this disease. I treat most of my patients who have PBC with 900 to 1,200 mg/day (3 to 4 capsules/day) of UDCA. Although UDCA is an expensive drug, a recent study has shown that patients who take this medicine have a lower incidence of major complications such as esophageal varices than patients who do not take it. Since treatment with UDCA can reduce the risk of such complications, it ultimately may lower medical costs.

Colchicine, a medicine that has been used for centuries to treat gout, also appears to be helpful in slowing the progression of PBC. Both UDCA and colchicine can be taken together. Recently, promising results were reported from a trial in which a combination of prednisone, azothioprine, and UDCA were used. The results of ongoing studies are awaited. Finally, recent studies have indicated that treatment with low doses of methotrexate, alone or in combination with other agents such as UDCA, may benefit some patients with PBC. Research into the use of this drug for PBC is ongoing.

TREATMENT OF SYMPTOMS

In addition to medications to slow down the progression of PBC, your physician also can recommend various treatments to relieve the symptoms of this disease.

Itching

If you have PBC, you probably won't be mistaken for the young belle of old Natchez, because chances are very good that you will be able to stop the itching (pruritis).

REMEDIES FOR OCCASIONAL ITCHING. If you have a mild case of pruritis, you may find that warm baths, emollients, alcohol sponges, and antihistamines such as benadryl provide some relief.

CHOLESTYRAMINE. If your itching is more severe and even debilitating, though, these remedies are usually not effective. In this case, I usually prescribe from 4 to 16 grams per day of a very effective drug called cholestyramine. This medication generally is taken with meals. Three to four days after treatment has begun, you probably will see some improvement.

If your doctor recommends that you take cholestyramine, which comes in a powder form, there are a few things that you should be aware of. First of all, it doesn't taste very good, so you should mix it with applesauce or fruit juice to make it palatable. This drug also can make you constipated, so your doctor may recommend that you take laxatives. Finally, cholestyramine can interact poorly with other medicines, including digoxin, warfarin, propranolol, and thiazide diuretics, so if you are taking any of these (or any other drugs) you should be sure to take the cholestyramine by itself at least a couple of hours before or after you take other medicines.

COLESTIPOL. Like cholestyramine, another drug known as colestipol can be very effective at stopping the itching associated with PBC. It's similar to cholestyramine in that it isn't very tasty, though, so if your doctor recommends that you try this medicine, you may want to have "a spoonful of sugar" nearby when you take it.

OTHER MEDICATIONS. If your itching is not alleviated by cholestyramine or colestipol, or if you are not able to tolerate them, other medications are available. These drugs include rifampin, cimetidine, phenobarbital, and morphine (opioid) antagonists such as naloxone, nalmefene, and naltrexone. Some of these opioid antagonists are still in clinical trials, but they may prove to be very effective in treating this symptom.

PHOTOTHERAPY. In addition to drug therapy for chronic itching, we sometimes refer patients with PBC to a dermatologist for phototherapy with ultraviolet B (UVB) light.

PLASMAPHERESIS. Another technique that sometimes is used to relieve the itching of PBC is known as plasmapheresis. This method involves drawing blood, removing the fluid called plasma from it, and then reinfusing the blood (sometimes after new "fresh frozen" plasma or a protein called albumin has been added). This expensive technique may be used as a "last resort" option if no other methods have worked. It has been used with good success in people with PBC who are waiting for liver transplants and suffer from truly unbearable itching.

LIVER TRANSPLANTATION. Finally, for the most severe and debilitating cases of itching associated with PBC, a liver transplant may be necessary. I'll talk more about this option later in this chapter.

Vitamin and Mineral Deficiencies

If PBC alters your body's ability to absorb fat, you may develop certain health problems related to malabsorption of fat-soluble vitamins (such as vitamins A, D, and K) and calcium. These conditions include night blindness and difficulty with dark adaption (vitamin A deficiency); bone pain and fractures (vitamin D and calcium deficiency); and nosebleeds, bleeding gums, and bruising (vitamin K deficiency).

To make up for these nutritional deficiencies, your physician will likely recommend that you take:

- Vitamin A—10,000 to 25,000 international units (IU)/day
- Vitamin D—1,000 IU/day;
- Vitamin K—3 to 5 mg by injection daily for three days
- Calcium—1,500 mg/day.

Diarrhea and Weight Loss

Problems with fat malabsorption also can cause diarrhea and weight loss. If you have these symptoms, I recommend that you restrict your dietary fat. Medium-chain triglyceride (MCT) oil also can be added to your diet to provide well-tolerated extra calories. If, despite these measures, diarrhea persists, it's possible that you have an associated deficiency of pancreatic enzymes. This insufficiency can be treated easily by taking pancreatic enzyme supplements (in the form of tablets) when you eat.

TREATMENT OF RELATED DISORDERS

Several other disorders have been known to occur with PBC, and you may need to be treated for them as well. These health problems include autoimmune conditions, gallstones, metabolic bone disease, cholesterol deposits in the skin, iron deficiency anemia, CRST syndrome, and dermatomyositis.

Autoimmune Conditions

As I mentioned earlier, hypothyroidism and dry gland syndrome are autoimmune disorders that sometimes coexist with PBC.

HYPOTHYROIDISM. If you have PBC, there is an estimated 20 percent chance that you also will have hypothyroidism (an underactive thyroid condition) or that you will develop this condition. Your doctor can diagnose hypothyroidism, which can cause fatigue, dry skin, and weight gain, by looking at certain thyroid hormone levels in your blood. If the results of these simple tests are abnormal, your physician can prescribe thyroid hormone replacement drug therapy. With such treatment, you may experience significant and indeed very gratifying relief of your hypothyroid symptoms.

DRY GLAND SYNDROME. If you experience dry gland syndrome along with your PBC, artificial tears can make your eyes feel better. Taking tablets of a drug called pilocarpine (Salagen) and drinking plenty of fluids can help if you have a dry mouth. Sugarless candies or mouth sprays also may be used to keep your mouth moist. I usually tell my patients who suffer from this condition to sit up and "chase" any medication that they take with lots of water, because if a pill gets lodged in the esophagus (this is called "pill esophagitis"), it can produce severe injury and inflammation.

Gallstones

Having PBC also carries with it a 30 to 40 percent risk of developing gallstones. Most often gallstones do not produce symptoms, and thus no treatment is required. However, if you develop symptoms (such as upper abdominal pain) or complications of gallstones (such as inflammation of the gallbladder or pancreas), you will likely need a surgical procedure called laparoscopic cholecystectomy to remove your gallbladder.

Metabolic Bone Disease

Another condition associated with PBC is metabolic bone disease (also known as hepatic osteodystrophy). We don't know what causes this condition, which can affect both men and women. (Women can develop this problem before, during, or after menopause.) Metabolic bone disease may be painful and can lead to hairline rib and vertebral fractures.

If you have PBC you have about a 25 percent chance of developing a form of metabolic bone disease, osteoporosis, which involves significant bone loss. The other form of this disease, osteomalacia, causes softening of the bones because of a loss of minerals. This disorder is less common, perhaps because of the widespread use of vitamin D supplements in milk and other common staples of the American diet. I recommend that all of my patients with PBC have their bone density checked when their PBC is diagnosed and then every couple of years. Bone density measurements can be determined by painless radiographic scanning techniques such as computed tomography (CT) and a new method called dual-energy X-ray absorptiometry, or DEXA.

If such tests reveal significant bone loss, you may wish to see a specialist in bone and mineral metabolism, although many internists are also well versed in this field, and they can offer you expert advice and management. You may be advised to take medications such as biphisphonates (e.g., etidronate) to prevent further bone loss. I also recommend that patients with PBC take supplements of 1,000 international units of vitamin D and 1,500 mg of calcium every day.

Many physicians are concerned about giving estrogen medications to people with liver disease because very rarely they can cause liver problems such as jaundice, and long-term use can (extremely rarely) lead to the development of a benign liver tumor (hepatic adenoma; see pages 221–223). However, I believe that by and large they are safe, and they can slow down the rate of bone loss. If you have PBC you should not take corticosteroids, however, because they can worsen your osteoporosis.

For severe osteoporosis with PBC, the definitive treatment is a liver transplant, which is described in detail in chapter 13. Although this operation eventually can improve bone mineral density, bed rest and the use of corticosteroids after the liver transplant may make the osteoporosis worse for the first six months. One year after the transplant, however, bone mineral density should begin to increase, and the risk of bone fractures should decrease. Calcium supplements are especially important during this period of bone formation.

Cholesterol Deposits in the Skin

As I mentioned earlier, the high level of cholesterol often associated with PBC can lead to deposits of this substance in your skin. These deposits sometimes create somewhat cosmetically disfiguring and rarely painful bumps called xanthelasmas (or xanthomas) on the hands, soles, elbows, knees, ankles, wrists, back, chest, or buttocks. If you have PBC, your risk of having these lesions is less than 10 percent; your risk is highest if you have advanced and untreated PBC.

Cholesterol deposits also may appear on your eyelids, where they can cause yellowish growths. These growths often return rapidly if they are excised, hence I don't recommend surgical removal. However, if your PBC is treated by other methods (such as with cholestyramine), the resulting lower level of cholesterol in your body may cause these fatty deposits to gradually go away.

Rarely, painful xanthomas or xanthelasmas can infiltrate the nerves and produce distressing symptoms. Plasmapheresis, the expensive blood removal and replacement procedure that I described earlier, is occasionally used to treat these painful cholesterol deposits. This procedure often needs to be repeated every few weeks until the blood cholesterol level normalizes, at which point the xanthomas will begin to disappear.

Iron Deficiency Anemia

Another disorder sometimes associated with PBC is iron deficiency anemia, a deficiency of red blood cells most often due to gastrointestinal blood loss. Less often, this type of anemia is caused by a coexisting but separate disease called celiac sprue (or gluten-sensitive enteropathy).

If your iron deficiency anemia is due to gastrointestinal blood loss, your gastroenterologist or hepatologist should be able to determine the exact cause of this bleeding. You may have obvious bleeding from ruptured engorged veins called varices in your esophagus (see chapter 9), or you may have more subtle bleeding due to a condition called congestive gastropathy, or congestion of the lining of the stomach, caused by increased pressure in your portal veins (the veins that carry blood from the stomach, spleen, and intestines to the liver). Your liver specialist will be able to manage these bleeding problems accordingly.

If celiac sprue is the cause of your iron deficiency, eating wheat, barley, or rye—common food items!—may damage your small intestine (small bowel). This injury can cause diarrhea and decreased absorption of nutrients such as iron from part of the small intestine. We recommend a special gluten-free diet for patients with this condition.

CRST Syndrome

CRST syndrome is a constellation of symptoms that includes: *calcinosis cutis* (calcium, rather than cholesterol, deposits in the skin), *Raynaud's phenomenon* (pain in the fingers and toes that may be caused by cold or emotional stress), *sclerodactyly* (hardening or thickening of the skin on the fingers and toes), and *telangiectasia* ("spider" veins, or small red lesions on the skin). If you have Raynaud's disease, your liver specialist may prescribe drugs called calcium channel blockers for you. For sclerodactyly, moisturizers for the thickened skin may be beneficial. If this disorder causes skin ulcers that become infected, your doctor may prescribe antibiotics.

Dermatomyositis

Dermatomyositis is skin inflammation that may cause swelling of the eyelids and a rash on the eyelids, forehead, neck, shoulders, trunk, and arms. In general, if these symptoms are severe or refractory (that is, if they do not respond to initial medical treatment with drugs such as steroids), I recommend that such patients see a rheumatologist, a specialist most familiar with treating painful or inflamed joints or muscles.

LIVER TRANSPLANTATION

Liver transplantation is the definitive treatment for people with end-stage PBC who have liver failure, or severe liver disease that has led to conditions such as progressive jaundice, intolerable itching, bleeding esophageal varices, or incapacitating mental changes (encephalopathy). If performed at an appropriate time, this operation can be quite successful. In fact, for patients with PBC, the one-year survival rate after liver transplantation is better than 80 percent. After this major operation (which is described in more detail in chapter 13), patients must have long-term treatment with medicines called immunosuppressants to prevent rejection of the new liver.

Recurrence of PBC in the donor or "new" organ may occur, although it's difficult to distinguish disease recurrence from the body's ongoing attempts to reject the new liver. In both cases, there is bile duct damage. Thus, if a patient who has had a liver transplant for PBC begins to have abnormal liver function (blood) test results, a biopsy of the liver will be done. Then the patient's hepatologist and a liver pathologist must evaluate many factors, including the biopsy results and the amount of immunosuppressants that the patient has been taking, before deciding on a plan of treatment.

SUMMARY

If you have PBC, you may wish to ask your physician the following questions:

1. What treatment do you recommend for the itching related to PBC?
2. Do I have a coexisting thyroid condition?

3. If my cholesterol level is high, is it because of "good" cholesterol that is not dangerous to my heart?
4. Should I be vaccinated against the hepatitis A or B viruses?
5. Do I have osteoporosis? What preventive or corrective actions should I take?
6. Do I have esophageal varices? If so, should I take medicine to decrease the risk of variceal bleeding?
7. Will you perform periodic tests to screen for liver cancer?

As you clarify these issues with your doctor and embark on a satisfactory plan to manage your illness, you should be encouraged to know that dedicated scientists are working to bring to light a greater understanding of what causes PBC, and hopefully better treatments for this condition will be available in the near future.

11

Iron Overload Disorders

I recently moved from San Francisco to Cambridge, Massachu-setts, to work for a small nonprofit organization, and for the most part things have been going very well. In my free time I've been soaking up Boston's history, spending more money than I should in bookstores, and running by the Charles River every morning before work. Even though I'm healthy—I take vitamins, and I work out every day —I thought it would be a good idea to find a doctor here, so I made an appointment to see a physician who was recommended to me by a colleague.

I had a normal checkup with my new doctor, and she asked me to have blood drawn for some routine tests. A few days later, she called to tell me that I may have an "iron overload" disorder. I'm going back to see her for more tests on Friday, and I have a whole list of questions to ask her. For instance, I wonder how I could have too much iron in my body if I don't eat red meat. Is it because I eat a lot of spinach? I'm also wondering if my multi-vitamins, which contain iron, could be responsible for this problem.

She mentioned that it was important to look into this possible iron overload disease because it may cause liver or heart prob-lems. It sounds a little scary. When I asked about treatment, she said something about phlebotomy, or "bloodletting." It really sounds medieval. I wonder if it works.

—IRENE KEELEY, age forty-three

Iron is an essential mineral for the proper functioning of the body. You've probably heard of iron deficiency anemia, a common condition that may be caused by gastrointestinal blood loss, heavy menstrual periods, or, in some parts of the world, hookworm infestations. Untreated, this type of anemia can cause severe fatigue and even a form of heart failure. The converse—that is, too much iron—can be harmful too, because the body can't get rid of excess amounts of this metallic element. In a unique iron overload disorder, extraordinary amounts of iron are absorbed from the intestines and then deposited throughout the body, where they can damage many different organs.

In the pancreas, an accumulation of iron can result in diabetes. In the pituitary gland, it can trigger endocrine problems, and in the heart muscle, too much iron can cause abnormal heart rhythms (arrhythmias), heart failure, and even death. Indeed, as Dame Sheila Sherlock, one of the world's most eminent liver specialists, once wrote, "The iron heart is a weak one."

Some of the most severe effects of iron overload occur in the liver, where deposits of this mineral can lead to an increase in fibrous tissue (fibrosis) and scarring (cirrhosis). Mild to moderate iron overload in this organ may be a consequence of alcoholic cirrhosis, chronic infection with the hepatitis C virus, or a condition called porphyria cutanea tarda (see page 210).

People with certain kinds of anemia and individuals who have received multiple blood transfusions also may develop iron overload. This disorder also can occur after a surgical procedure known as a portocaval shunt, which was performed commonly decades ago to treat bleeding veins (varices) in the esophagus. Iron overload on rare occasions may be caused by ingestion of food or beer that was fermented in iron pots. I'll tell you more about these causes later on. The main focus of this chapter is an inherited form of iron overload, idiopathic genetic hemochromatosis, which is the most common genetic disorder known to man.

IDIOPATHIC GENETIC HEMOCHROMATOSIS

ARE YOU AT RISK?

Not too long ago we considered idiopathic genetic hemochromatosis, or simply "hemochromatosis," to be a very rare disorder, but now we know that in Caucasians of northern European descent it is the most common inherited disorder. In fact, this disease, which affects more than 1 million Americans, is 5 to 10 times more common than cystic fibrosis.

A far greater number of people carry the gene for this disease. In August 1996 scientists discovered the gene that's responsible for hereditary hemochromatosis (the "HFE gene"). This genetic mutation probably arose many eons ago in a Celtic ancestor, because the incidence of this disease is highest in places where there are many people of Celtic descent. For instance, roughly 1 in 300 people in Brittany, France; Brisbane, Australia; Boston, Massachusetts; and Salt Lake City, Utah, have hemochromatosis. Although studies have elucidated the high prevalence of hemochromatosis in the white Caucasian population of Irish descent, there appear to be far fewer cases of this disorder among Asian Americans and African Americans.

SYMPTOMS

Hemochromatosis is present at birth, but generally it is "silent" early in its course, and most often it doesn't create noticeable symptoms until the middle of life (ages forty to sixty). If you have hemochromatosis, you may have no symptoms at all, or you may have mild to moderate abdominal pain or discomfort, weakness, lethargy, impotence, or weight loss.

RELATED DISORDERS

In addition to the symptoms mentioned above, you also may have symptoms of other conditions that can be associated with hemochromatosis, such as diabetes, arthritis, endocrine disorders, heart failure, and liver scarring (cirrhosis).

DIABETES. In 1935, Dr. Sheldon in England first described the classic triad of hemochromatosis: an enlarged liver, increased skin pigmentation, and diabetes mellitus, a disorder of carbohydrate metabolism. Indeed, for many decades hemochromatosis was called "bronzed diabetes," because people with this condition often had both diabetes and a peculiar bronze discoloration of the skin. These days, better screening for hemochromatosis means that fewer people now have diabetes when their iron overload disorder is diagnosed. If your iron overload disorder was diagnosed early, and you haven't developed cirrhosis, your risk of having diabetes is as low as 20 percent. If you do have advanced disease, though, your chance of having diabetes is as high as 70 percent.

Symptoms of diabetes mellitus that you should watch for include increased thirst, hunger, and weight loss. Your doctor can diagnose this condition by blood tests.

ARTHRITIS. Iron deposits can also affect the joints, and recent studies suggest that up to 15 percent of people who have hemochromatosis also have a particular form of arthritis called "pseudogout." Like gout, pseudogout causes painful inflammation of the joints. If your physician suspects that you may have this type of arthritis, she may take X-ray films of your joints and a sample of the joint fluid to study under the microscope. She will be looking for particular crystals in the fluid that are diagnostic of pseudogout.

ENDOCRINE DISORDERS. In addition to iron deposits in your liver, pancreas, and joints, excessive amounts of iron also can build up in your pituitary gland and cause endocrine disorders that may lead to a loss of libido, impotence in men, and early menopause in women.

INFECTIONS. Patients with hemochromatosis also have a greater likelihood of acquiring certain unusual bacterial infections such as *Yersinia enterocolitica,* which can cause diarrhea, arthritis, and abdominal discomfort. This constellation of symptoms can resemble an inflammatory intestinal disorder known as Crohn's disease. Investigators also have discovered a link between hemochromatosis and a higher than usual incidence of infections with *Listeria monocytogenes, E. coli,* and *Candida.*

HEART PROBLEMS. When iron is deposited in the heart muscle, or myocardium, the heart muscle doesn't pump very well, and this can lead to a form of heart failure called cardiomyopathy. This condition can lead to fluid retention, so if you have this disorder, your ankles may swell. You also may have difficulty breathing.

Excess amounts of iron in the heart also can cause potentially serious abnormal heart rhythms known as arrhythmias. Classic symptoms of an irregular heartbeat can include weakness, fatigue, lightheadedness, palpitations, chest pressure, nausea, and shortness of breath.

CIRRHOSIS. Roughly 5 percent of people who are diagnosed with hemochromatosis today have advanced liver disease. That is, they have cirrhosis of the liver with the potential for all of its attendant complications, including a swollen, fluid-filled abdomen (ascites) and engorged veins called varices in the esophagus. If your disease is severe, you may feel fatigued and nauseated, and you may have lost your appetite. You also may have itchy skin, a yellowish cast to your skin and the whites of your eyes (jaundice), and a tendency to bleed easily. Cirrhosis and its complications are described more fully in chapter 9.

DIAGNOSIS

Early detection of hemochromatosis through a simple blood test and early treatment are extremely important, because even if you have no symptoms, iron absorption often continues with each passing day, week, and month until there are high concentrations of iron in your liver that can lead to severe fibrosis and cirrhosis.

Half a century ago, most people were not diagnosed with hemochromatosis until they were between fifty and sixty years of age, when they first had symptoms of this disorder. Often they survived at most five years after their disease was recognized because they succumbed to the complications of cirrhosis (including primary liver cancer, which was responsible for 75 percent of deaths) or to complications of diabetes or heart failure.

In recent years, though, the clinical landscape has changed tremendously. A quarter century ago, 25 to 50 percent of people who were newly diagnosed with this disease had no symptoms. Today we have a better appreciation of how common this disorder is, though, and we are screening for it more often and detecting it at an earlier stage, when life-saving treatment can be started. As a result, now more than 75 percent of people diagnosed with hemochromatosis don't have symptoms. They tend to be younger and have less iron accumulation than people with iron overload disorders in the past, so they are also less likely to have significant damage to many organs, and their prospects for long-term survival are better than ever.

SCREENING

> *The prevention and control of hereditary hemochromatosis is*
> *an achievable goal and an important chronic disease prevention*
> *opportunity.*
> —U.S. CENTERS FOR DISEASE CONTROL AND PREVENTION,
> *Guidelines for Hereditary Hemochromatosis,* 1998

In spite of these strides, it's still not unusual for a delayed diagnosis to occur up to five to ten years after a person first experiences symptoms, and occasionally patients have to see several physicians before their iron overload condition is diagnosed. Such delays wouldn't happen if screening for hemochromatosis were universal. I believe that testing for hemochromatosis fulfills the four ideal requisites for screening large populations:

1. It's a common disorder.
2. The screening test (a blood test called iron saturation) is simple and not that expensive.
3. If we diagnose this disorder at an early stage (before people have developed diabetes mellitus or cirrhosis), and if treatment is started early in the course of the disease, they will remain healthy. In fact, their life expectancy will be the same as those of people of the same gender and age who do not have this disease.
4. Once a doctor diagnoses hemochromatosis in one person, she can screen that person's siblings and, at the right age, his children (I recommend screening in general after the age of ten years). Thus, screening just one person for hemochromatosis may, in the end, have a huge impact on the lives of several individuals.

My patient Irene learned that she had genetic hemochromatosis because of routine screening. She went to visit her new primary care physician for a physical, and her examination was completely normal. Irene then had her blood drawn, and as part of a comprehensive evaluation her doctor sent off a blood sample to a laboratory for tests called iron studies. The results of these tests turned out to be very abnormal, and they raised the possibility of hemochromatosis.

Irene's physician called me one morning to discuss this possible diagnosis. She said that Irene did not have any symptoms or a history of liver disease, and there was no history of liver disease in her family. I asked if she was taking a multivitamin, and it turned out that she was taking one that contained iron.

Irene's doctor then asked Irene to stop taking this supplement, but when her iron saturation blood test was repeated one month later, it showed that her iron level was still markedly abnormal. (The normal level is around 30 percent, and Irene's level was 68 percent.) This test result suggested a diagnosis of hemochromatosis.

When Irene's doctor referred her to me, I ascertained that she had mild enlargement of the liver, and subsequently I performed a liver biopsy to obtain a small sample of liver tissue for testing. I suspected that Irene had hemochromatosis, so I obtained an extra "core" of tissue and sent it to a specialized laboratory. After a few days, I received the results from the laboratory with a measurement of the amount of iron in the liver tissue. We then used a formula that calculates what is known as the hepatic iron concentration index. A level of 1.9 or greater is virtually diagnostic of hemochromatosis. Irene's hepatic concentration index was 2.8, so she definitely had this iron overload disorder. The good news, though, was that the liver biopsy did not show liver scarring, or cirrhosis. Irene then began to undergo treatment with a procedure called phlebotomy (which I'll discuss later on in this chapter), and she has since done very well.

Unlike Irene, who was fortunate to be screened for hemochromatosis and began treatment early enough to prevent major damage to her liver, another patient of mine was not diagnosed with this disorder in time to stop the progression of this disease to cirrhosis. Dan was fifty years old when he went to see his primary care doctor for an annual physical. Nothing looked abnormal during his physical examination, but a comprehensive battery of blood tests showed that Dan had mild elevations in levels of two liver enzymes called alanine transaminase (ALT) and aspartate transaminase (AST). These enzymes, which are released by damaged liver cells, can be elevated with a number of different liver disorders. At this time, Dan's doctor did not perform blood tests called iron studies, so there was no attempt to test for hemochromatosis.

Dan's doctor suspected that these abnormal ALT and AST results were related to alcohol consumption, because patients with alcoholic liver disease often have elevated liver enzyme levels. When she asked Dan about his alcohol consumption, he told her that he drank one or two glasses of wine three to four times per week. He also noted that his father drank "quite a bit" and died at the age of sixty-three of "some kind of unusual infection." She recommended that he stop drinking alcohol and asked that he return for further blood tests after one month.

The next set of blood tests showed that although there was some improvement, Dan's ALT and AST levels were still above normal. His doctor then tested Dan's blood to determine whether or not he might have chronic viral hepatitis B or C (which also could cause these abnormal levels), but these tests were negative. Dan's physician thus presumed that Dan's abnormal liver enzyme results were related to alcohol, and over the next several years, during annual visits, she reminded him that he shouldn't drink. No iron studies were done, however.

Eight years later, when he was fifty-eight, Dan noticed that he was losing weight, and he wondered why he always felt thirsty. He went back to his doctor, and after doing some tests, she told him that he had diabetes mellitus. She then referred Dan to an endocrinologist, who found that Dan had a mildly enlarged liver, "spider" veins, and small testes— potential signs of cirrhosis. It was the endocrinologist who for the first time raised the possibility that Dan might have hemochromatosis.

Dan subsequently was referred to me. His blood was drawn to see if he had abnormal iron indices, and the results were markedly abnormal. Dan's iron saturation was 88 percent (we're suspicious of iron overload once this level gets above 50 percent), and his serum ferritin level was greater than 1,000 nanograms per milliliter (ng/ml; the normal range is 20–200 ng/ml for men and 10–150 ng/ml for women). I then did a liver biopsy that revealed scarring (cirrhosis) as well as tremendous deposits of iron in Dan's liver cells. I also sent a piece of the biopsy specimen to a specialized lab (as we had done for Irene) for calculation of the hepatic iron concentration index, which turned out to be 5.8—very high. Dan then had a procedure called an upper GI endoscopy that showed that he already had developed a potentially serious complication from his cirrhosis: moderate-size, engorged veins (varices) in his esophagus.

I was concerned that Dan's liver disease may have progressed even further, to primary hepatocellular carcinoma (primary cancer arising within the liver), so we also did an ultrasound scan of his liver, but fortunately we found no tumor. A blood test called alpha-fetoprotein (AFP) used to detect liver cancer was also normal, and I was relieved to assure Dan that he did not have liver cancer. He was relieved, too, but he had many questions about his hemochromatosis and cirrhosis. Most particularly, he wanted to know if his father might have had the same condition. He also asked if his condition could have been diagnosed earlier.

I told him that indeed, his father may very well have had idiopathic genetic hemochromatosis that led to cirrhosis of the liver. The fact that Dan's father drank and died of cirrhosis was not proof that alcohol caused his cirrhosis. Likewise, by assuming that Dan's abnormal test results were due to alcohol consumption, his primary care physician had overlooked a potentially treatable cause of his liver disease—iron overload. If she had done iron studies to look for hemochromatosis early on, she may have been able to diagnose and treat his iron overload, and hence spare him from the diabetes and cirrhosis that subsequently ensued.

PHYSICAL EXAMINATION. If you have hemochromatosis, when you visit your doctor you may (like Irene) have a completely normal physical examination, or your physician may find that (like Dan) you have signs of more advanced disease. These signs may include an enlarged liver, increased skin pigmentation, shrunken testes, features of chronic liver disease (such as red "spider" veins or red palms), or features of heart failure.

LABORATORY TESTS. Regardless of whether or not your physical examination is normal, your doctor may suspect that you have a liver problem if you have abnormal results on routine blood tests that often are referred to as liver function tests (LFTs). LFTs include the liver enzymes (ALT, AST, and another enzyme called alkaline phosphatase); prothrombin time (a measure of your blood's clotting ability); bilirubin (a bile pigment); and a protein called albumin. These tests are described in more detail in chapter 2.

We don't use liver enzyme tests to screen for hemochromatosis, because these levels are abnormal in only about half of people with this disorder. If your results are abnormal, then, your physician will need to do other tests to figure out the exact reason.

Other blood tests sometimes called iron studies *can* be very suggestive of hemochromatosis, and these should be used as screening tests. The most common ones are serum iron, total iron-binding capacity (TIBC), and serum ferritin. These tests reflect abnormal iron stores in the body, so if these results are abnormal and there is no other explanation (for instance, you're not taking a multivitamin that contains iron), you probably have an iron overload disorder.

Today good primary care physicians are checking iron study tests routinely (often as part of a patient's first visit) to look for hemochromatosis. Here's a little more information about these tests:

- **Serum ferritin.** Ferritin is a protein that stores iron in the liver. An elevated ferritin level *may* indicate that you have iron overload, but we don't use the ferritin level alone as a screening test for hemochromatosis, because it can be normal in people with this disorder. Serum ferritin also may be elevated with alcoholic liver disease, nonalcoholic steatohepatitis (NASH; see chapter 8), Hodgkin's lymphoma, rheumatoid arthritis, and kidney failure.
- **Serum iron concentration and percent transferrin saturation.** These two levels usually are elevated abnormally in people with hemochromatosis.
- **C-282-Y mutation test.** This blood test looks for a particular genetic mutation (called c-282-Y); it can be done for approximately $200 to $250. However, in 1997 an expert panel convened by the United States Centers for Disease Control (CDC) and the National Human Genome Institute (NHGI) recommended against the use of this genetic screening test because in many cases people who have

the gene for hemochromatosis do not have the illness. The panel expressed concern that once this genetic testing is done and the result goes into a person's medical record, he or she may have difficulty getting health or life insurance later on. In addition, not all individuals who have the genetic mutation actually have or develop excessive iron accumulation in vital organs such as the liver, heart, or pancreas.

IMAGING STUDIES. When I told Dan that he had genetic hemochromatosis with cirrhosis, he asked me whether he should have had a CAT scan at some point over the years and whether or not such a test would have shown that he had iron overload. These were very good questions! Both a computed axial tomographic (CAT, or simply CT) scan and magnetic resonance imaging (MRI) may show an increased density of the liver (which would suggest iron overload). However, findings from these imaging scans can be normal in patients with hemochromatosis. Furthermore, these studies may not necessarily show whether or not you have cirrhosis.

LIVER BIOPSY. A liver biopsy remains the gold standard for the diagnosis of iron overload. In this simple procedure, which usually is done on an outpatient basis, a small needle is used to obtain a bit of liver tissue for analysis under the microscope (see chapter 2). As I mentioned earlier, a sample of liver tissue obtained from a biopsy can be sent to a special laboratory for calculation of the hepatic iron concentration index. A hepatic iron concentration index level greater than 1.9 is diagnostic of hemochromatosis. A biopsy is also useful for determining the severity of your disease—that is, whether or not you have liver scarring (cirrhosis).

If a needle (also called a percutaneous) biopsy cannot be done because your abdomen is full of fluid (because of a complication of cirrhosis known as ascites) or because you have a significant bleeding tendency—or if you refuse to have a liver biopsy—your physician might do a CT or MRI scan instead, but these tests will not provide as much useful diagnostic information as a liver biopsy. Only by looking at the liver cells under a microscope can a physician determine exactly how excessive deposits of iron have affected your liver.

A major reason for doing the liver biopsy is to see if cirrhosis has developed. Recent studies suggest that if the patient is younger than age forty, the liver is not enlarged, the AST level in the blood is normal, and the serum ferritin is less than 1,000 ng/ml, then it is very unlikely that the patient will have cirrhosis. In patients who fulfill these criteria, one could avoid liver biopsy and begin treatment.

OTHER DIAGNOSTIC TESTS AND PROCEDURES. In addition to tests to confirm a diagnosis of iron overload and to ascertain how severe your condition is, your doctor also will have you undergo tests to look for other coexisting problems and complications.

- **Endoscopy.** If your hemochromatosis has caused cirrhosis, you should be screened for enlarged veins (varices) in your esophagus that, if present, may rupture and bleed. This test generally is done during an outpatient procedure called endoscopy (see chapter 9). If your physician finds that you do have esophageal varices, he or she may prescribe a medicine belonging to a class of drugs called beta blockers to decrease the chance of bleeding.
- **Tests for viral hepatitis A and B infections.** With a simple blood test, your doctor can determine whether or not you are at risk for acquiring the hepatitis A or B viruses. If you are at risk, effective vaccines are available to protect you from infection (these viral illnesses, "superimposed" on any other liver disease, including hemochromatosis, can make you very sick).

PRIMARY LIVER CANCER. If you don't have cirrhosis, your risk of having liver cancer as a complication of hemochromatosis is practically nonexistent! With the first patient mentioned in this chapter, Irene, we weren't concerned about liver cancer, because she did not have cirrhosis. If your hemochromatosis has evolved into cirrhosis, though, your risk of primary cancer of the liver (also known as primary hepatocellular carcinoma) is quite high—on the order of 25 percent. This is another reason why it's very important to diagnose hemochromatosis and to start treatment at an early stage of the disease.

As we did for Dan, your doctor can perform periodic alpha-fetoprotein (AFP) blood tests (every four months) and radiographic imaging tests such as an ultrasound or CAT scan (approximately every six months) to look for a liver tumor. If a tumor is caught at an early stage, a surgeon will be able to remove it in a procedure called a hepatectomy. The symptoms, diagnosis, and treatment of liver cancer are described in detail in chapter 12.

TREATMENT

PHLEBOTOMY. Although a "bloodletting," or phlebotomy, procedure sounds medieval, it remains the treatment of choice. This simple procedure usually involves going to a phlebotomy laboratory to have 1 to 2 units of blood drawn per week.

The procedure. You may be wondering what you might expect when you go to have your blood drawn. First of all, when you get to the phlebotomy lab, you probably will be encouraged to have something to eat and drink before this procedure. Next, you will have a blood test to check your level of hemoglobin (the part of the red blood cells that carries oxygen). Then you will have a brief interview with a staff member. Your blood will be drawn intravenously, and you'll be observed for a while after the procedure. After you have had something to eat or drink, you'll be free to leave. The entire visit may last up to an hour, although the actual blood drawing usually takes only minutes.

Side effects. Occasionally patients may experience side effects after phlebotomy. These include dizziness, headache, and bruising or swelling where the needle went into the arm. If you feel faint or dizzy, you may be advised to lie down or sit with your head between your knees. To replace some of the fluid that you've lost during this procedure, it's also helpful to drink an extra couple of glasses of fluid during the four hours after phlebotomy. You probably will be given an elastic bandage after the needle has been taken out of your arm. You should keep this bandage dry, and you can remove it after a few hours. If you have bleeding from the puncture site, apply pressure to the bleeding area and raise your arm until the bleeding stops. Notify your doctor if there is any unusual bleeding, bruising, or swelling at this site.

You don't necessarily need to be accompanied by a friend or family member, but if you are concerned about feeling faint or dizzy afterward, you may want to have someone with you. You most likely will be advised not to exercise strenuously for four to six hours after phlebotomy.

How often will this procedure be necessary? Each unit of blood that is removed contains 250 ml of iron. To remove 1 gram of iron, then, 4 units of blood must be taken. If the phlebotomist can remove 10 to 20 grams of extra iron over a number of months, and you don't become anemic, then you certainly have an iron overload disorder. Some of my patients have been adequately "de-ironed" by this method after 15 units of blood were removed, and for other patients we have had to remove 200 units of blood (so if they come for phlebotomy once a week, it takes two years). In healthy people, one can actually accelerate this process of iron removal by taking as many as 2 units of blood per week, but for practical purposes it usually ends up being 1 unit per week.

Irene was started on weekly phlebotomy, and every week a unit of blood was removed. After eighteen weeks, the blood tests showed that she was borderline iron deficient. At this point we stopped the weekly phlebotomies, and she is now on a maintenance phlebotomy regimen, which means that she comes in and has a unit of blood taken out every three months or so. This is to prevent reaccumulation of iron.

After you have been successfully "de-ironed," your underlying iron overload defect will remain, so excessive amounts of iron will continue to be absorbed and deposited in the organs and tissues of your body. Therefore, like Irene, you should continue maintenance phlebotomy sessions about once every three months.

With successful phlebotomy treatment, you could notice a dramatic increase in your energy and your general sense of well-being, you may gain weight, and your abdominal pain, if present, may disappear. This procedure also may improve the color of your skin and sometimes can be instrumental in improving certain health problems such as related heart failure and diabetes. However, phlebotomy will not affect gonadal failure or joint pain, and your risk of primary liver cancer will remain at 25 percent if you have developed cirrhosis. (In contrast, if you don't have cirrhosis, your risk of liver cancer remains at zero, and your life expectancy should be normal.)

Finally, you may wonder if phlebotomy can reverse your cirrhosis. Although this outcome can occur, the likelihood that it will is exceedingly rare.

DESFEROXYMINE. In special circumstances, if you cannot tolerate phlebotomy because of severe anemia (a deficiency of red blood cells), your doctor can give you a "chelating" medicine called desferoxymine. Right now patients are given desferoxymine by an infusion pump, but in the near future oral chelating medicines may become available.

OTHER RECOMMENDATIONS

When Irene first came to my office, she was a little anxious. She said, "Dr. Chopra, my internist said that I may have a condition called hemochromatosis. I know very little about it. Is it an inherited disorder? If so, should my younger sister be tested?" I told her that because this iron overload disorder is inherited, we do advise siblings and children of people with hemochromatosis to be screened for this disease.

Irene also asked me if I had any specific lifestyle recommendations in addition to her phlebotomy treatment. I answered that if you have advanced hemochromatosis, you must not drink any alcohol, because alcohol can accelerate the damage to your liver. I also recommended that she avoid large amounts of vitamin C, because this vitamin actually can increase the amount of iron that is absorbed through the gastrointestinal tract and can be damaging to the heart. On the other hand, a deficiency of vitamin C can interfere with the effectiveness of desferoxymine, so if you take this chelating agent, you should speak with your doctor about how much vitamin C is appropriate for you.

OTHER CAUSES OF IRON OVERLOAD

Although increased iron deposition in the liver is a hallmark of genetic hemochromatosis, high amounts of iron can be found in the liver with other, mostly noninherited conditions, too. Dietary factors, multiple blood transfusions, rare types of anemias (some are inherited), chronic infection with the hepatitis C virus, alcoholic liver disease, and a surgical procedure known as a portocaval shunt all may lead to this type of disorder, which is called secondary hemochromatosis.

DIET

It's possible to develop an iron overload disorder after taking iron supplements for long periods of time, and if you have a preexisting iron overload disorder, ingesting too much iron from multivitamins can exacerbate your condition. However, the iron absorption problems related to most cases of iron overload disorders are not caused by eating too many iron-rich foods (such as red meat and spinach).

The only exception that I can think of is an iron overload disorder known as Bantu siderosis. Many years ago, iron overload was documented in a tribe in sub-Saharan Africa known as the Bantus. They drank low-alcohol beer that was fermented in iron pots or steel drums. The iron leached into the beer, and members of the tribe may have ingested as much as 100 mg of iron daily from this beer. Similarly, Ethiopians have been known to develop iron overload disorders after eating porridge (called teff) that has been fermented in iron pots.

BLOOD TRANSFUSIONS

It's also possible to develop iron overload if you have received multiple blood transfusions.

CHRONIC HEPATITIS C VIRAL INFECTION

Some patients with hepatitis C viral infection have mildly increased levels of iron. Phlebotomy may be a useful adjunctive maneuver in the treatment of such patients (see chapter 6).

ALCOHOLIC LIVER DISEASE

If you have alcoholic liver disease (see chapter 8), you also may have iron overload, although generally your liver concentrations of this element will not be as high as those found in people with genetic hemochromatosis.

PORTOCAVAL SHUNTS

After a surgical procedure known as a portocaval shunt, which once was performed commonly for the treatment of variceal bleeding (see pages 167–69), a person may develop a mild iron overload disorder. This is called post-shunt iron overload.

Today, instead of shunts, newer techniques such as endoscopic band ligation are performed to stop variceal bleeding. By this method, the culprit varices in the foodpipe (esophagus) are literally tied off with rubber bands to stop the bleeding. Endoscopic band ligation and other procedures for the treatment of esophageal varices are described in more detail in chapter 9.

PORPHYRIA CUTANEA TARDA

Liver diseases and iron overload often coexist with a condition called porphyria cutanea tarda, which is caused by abnormalities in metabolism of a pigment called porphyrin. This condition can lead to lesions or scarring on sun-exposed areas of your skin. If you have this disorder, you should avoid direct sunlight, and you should not drink alcohol. Phlebotomy is usually helpful.

SUMMARY

In the last few years, we've made some strides in screening for iron overload disorders. The medical community needs to do this screening in a much more systematic and rigorous fashion so that we can diagnose patients at an early stage, before they have developed serious consequences such as severe liver scarring (cirrhosis) or diabetes.

My hope is that universal screening (in Caucasian individuals over the age of thirty years) soon will be adopted so that patients with this very manageable disorder can be identified and then treated at an early stage with complete and gratifying success.

12

....

Liver Tumors

What do you think of when you hear the words *liver tumor?* For many people, the first thing that comes to mind is cancer that spreads (metastasizes) from another part of the body—the lungs, breast, pancreas, stomach, or colon, for example—to the liver. Because of this large organ's very rich blood supply, cancer cells commonly migrate to it.

Sometimes, when these malignant cells find their way to the liver, we may discover a single metastatic lesion or a few small lesions clustered in one lobe of the liver. There may be no evidence of metastasis to other parts of the body. In such instances, the patient can be referred to a capable liver surgeon, who can remove that part of the liver via a procedure known as a partial hepatectomy.

This happens infrequently, though. Most patients whose cancer has spread to the liver really don't need the expertise of a liver specialist (a hepatologist), but rather a cancer specialist, or oncologist, whose task is to figure out where the tumor originated and then to direct the appropriate treatment, depending on the nature of the malignancy. The main focus of this chapter thus is not on cancer that has spread to the liver from another part of the body, but on tumors that arise within the liver itself.

But what exactly is a tumor? It's simply an abnormal mass of tissue that grows from already existing tissue and serves no useful function in the body. Like those that develop elsewhere, tumors that arise within the liver can be benign (noncancerous, nonspreading, and favorable in that they generally have a good outcome) or malignant (which means they can be progressive, they tend to spread, and, untreated, they can be fatal).

The most common benign tumors of the liver include hepatic hemangiomas, hepatic adenomas, and focal nodular hyperplasia. The major malignant tumor arising within the liver has several names, including primary liver cancer, primary hepatocellular carcinoma, and hepatoma. For simplicity's sake, I'll refer to these malignancies as hepatomas. In this chapter I'd like to tell you how these tumors come to clinical attention, how a liver specialist may determine what kind of tumors they are, and the different forms of treatment that are available.

HOW DO LIVER TUMORS COME TO LIGHT?

I was playing golf one afternoon, and on the fifteenth hole I suddenly had some pain on my right side, just below my right rib cage. It was very uncomfortable, but I managed to finish the round.

It went away a few hours later, and I thought I'd had a muscle spasm. Then a few days later, it came back—the same pain in the same place. And I began to have some nausea.

I saw my doctor, who did a complete physical exam and ordered blood tests; everything looked fine. He thought the pain might have been caused by a gallstone, so I had an ultrasound exam. That's when they found the mass in my liver.

CHANCE FINDING

Although tumors may come to light because they are producing symptoms, you may have no symptoms at all, and a tumor may appear as a total surprise when a radiologic test is done for some other reason. For example, if you have pelvic pain or blood in your urine, your doctor may order an ultrasound or computed axial tomographic (CAT) scan to look at the pelvic organs or the kidneys—and discover the liver lesion by chance. Sometimes these tumors are found when an ultrasound exam is done to look at the developing fetus in an apparently normal pregnancy.

Cancer Screening

For people with certain chronic liver diseases, we do recommend regular screening tests to look for liver tumors because such patients have a higher risk of developing a malignant cancer known as a hepatoma.

For instance, people with liver scarring (cirrhosis) caused by too much iron in the liver (hemochromatosis) and people who have chronic infection with the hepatitis B virus (HBV) or hepatitis C virus (HCV) often are screened every six months by an ultrasound exam of the liver. They also have a blood test called alpha-fetoprotein (AFP) every four to six months to ascertain if a malignant tumor might be developing. A significant increase in this protein level can suggest the presence of a hepatoma. With all of these conditions, the risk of developing hepatoma is highest if the liver disease has led to cirrhosis.

No matter how your liver tumor may have been discovered, it's likely that your primary care physician will refer you to a gastroenterologist or hepatologist who has substantial experience in taking care of patients with such a problem. Look for a medical center that has a skilled team of gastroenterologists, hepatologists, radiologists, surgeons, and liver oncologists. In many academic centers, such experts conduct weekly conferences to discuss the best treatment plan for patients with liver tumors.

Symptoms

You may first become aware of a liver tumor because you're having symptoms. These symptoms usually are nonspecific (which means that they could relate to many different illnesses): you may experience pain in the right upper part of your abdomen (which is where the liver is), jaundice, nausea, weakness, fatigue, loss of appetite, vomiting, or significant weight loss. If these vague symptoms persist or are bothersome, you will likely see your doctor, who will examine you and order blood tests and special liver imaging studies.

Liver cancer can also create more dramatic and specific symptoms that may lead the physician to target the liver as a source of the problem. Tumor growth can cause the abdomen to swell with fluid that accumulates around the liver and intestines (this is called ascites). Rising levels of bilirubin, a bile pigment in your blood, may make your skin and the whites of your eyes look yellow (jaundiced). In any of these instances, your doctor will likely request that you have an imaging study such as an ultrasound or a CAT scan, and this scan may show that you have a liver tumor.

WHAT KIND OF TUMOR DO YOU HAVE?

My doctor said that he'd refer me to a specialist. He told me that the fact that my blood tests were normal was reassuring. Still, the idea of having a liver tumor was absolutely terrifying. I couldn't rest until I knew whether or not it was malignant.

Quite often I see patients who have just learned from their primary care physician that they have a liver tumor. When they come to my office, they usually are quite alarmed and concerned that the lesion might be cancerous. They often ask whether there is any cure, and they wonder whether major surgery or a liver transplant might be necessary. To answer these important questions and to sort out exactly what kind of tumor we're dealing with, I take a very detailed history from the patient, perform a physical examination, and obtain certain blood tests. I also often do further radiologic tests.

HISTORY

Your medical history can provide your liver specialist with important clues about your liver mass. He or she may ask the following questions:

1. Do you have any symptoms?
2. Have you ever had any imaging studies done in the past? If you had an ultrasound for some other reason two or three years ago, for example, your physician can retrieve the scan and check whether the lesion was present at that time. If it was and the mass hasn't changed over the last few years, that's very comforting, because it's unlikely to be a malignant tumor.
3. Do you have cirrhosis? This is important because malignant tumors called hepatomas usually occur in patients who have this condition. But remember, not all patients with cirrhosis develop this type of tumor!
4. What is your family's medical history? Your liver specialist will want to know if anyone in your family has had any of the following:
   • Genetic hemochromatosis (a disorder in which too much iron is deposited in the liver)
   • Chronic infection with either the hepatitis B virus (HBV) or hepatitis C virus (HCV)
   • Hepatoma
   • Hereditary tyrosinema (a buildup of an amino acid called tyrosine that can lead to liver disease)

   If there is a family history of any of these disorders, one would be more concerned that the lesion could be malignant, because these conditions are all risk factors for hepatoma. Although hepatoma itself is not inherited genetically, some of these predisposing risk factors are.
5. Do you have any risk factors for having acquired HBV or HCV infection? These include accidentally sticking yourself with a contaminated syringe, having sex with a person infected with one of these viruses, getting a tattoo or acupuncture with unclean needles, and receiving blood or blood products before 1992 (see chapters 3–6).
6. What medicines or toxins have you been exposed to in the past? All of the following agents may contribute to the development of certain liver tumors: birth control pills; anabolic steroids (sometimes taken by athletes); alcohol; arsenic; vinyl chloride (a

chemical that's used in the rubber industry); thorotrast (a radioactive contrast material that once was used in radiologic imaging studies); and aflatoxin (a contaminant of corn, peanuts, and soybeans which is common in parts of Africa and Southeast Asia and in some of the drinking water in rural China).

PHYSICAL EXAMINATION

When your liver specialist examines you, he will be on the lookout for features of chronic liver diseases (such as cirrhosis) that may have predisposed you to the development of hepatoma. These features include either an enlarged or a shrunken liver, an enlarged spleen, and possibly certain skin (cutaneous) findings such as red palms or red spider veins.

LABORATORY TESTS

After your physical exam, in all likelihood you'll be asked to have blood drawn to look for a potential cause of your liver tumor (such as chronic HBV or HCV infection) as well as a "tumor marker" that may suggest the severity of your disease. These laboratory blood tests may or may not turn out to be informative or diagnostic:

- **Complete blood count (CBC).** Alterations in the CBC can be a clue to your doctor about the nature of your tumor. With benign tumors, the red blood count usually is normal, unless there has been bleeding that would bring the blood count down. On the other hand, if the tumor is malignant, a low red blood cell count (anemia) may be present. On rare occasions, a hepatoma can produce a hormone called erythropoietin, which is needed for the bone marrow to produce red blood cells. If a patient who was anemic (because of a condition such as cirrhosis) in the past suddenly is no longer anemic, it may be because a hepatoma is producing this hormone and causing increased red blood cell production.
- **Liver function profile.** Certain liver function tests (LFTs) often are normal or mildly elevated with benign tumors, but with malignant tumors (both those that arise within the liver and those that spread from elsewhere in the body) there are often abnormal

results. For example, a dramatic increase in an enzyme called alkaline phosphatase may be a clue to hepatoma. Striking increases in both the alkaline phosphatase level and the level of another enzyme called lactate dehydrogenase (LDH) could be due to metastatic liver disease.

- **Markers for HBV and HCV infection.** Specific blood tests will be done to see whether or not you are infected with one or both of these viruses (both of which can lead to cirrhosis and, in turn, to hepatoma).
- **Other specialized blood tests such as alpha-fetoprotein (AFP).** AFP, a protein that can be measured in the blood, is considered to be a "serum marker" for hepatoma. In the United States, it's found in high concentrations in the blood of more than 70 percent of patients with this type of tumor. However, benign disease (and pregnancy) also can cause these elevations, and people with malignancy can have normal AFP levels. It's best to discuss the results of these tests with your physician.

RADIOLOGIC TESTS

By this point, in addition to having a physical exam and a battery of blood tests, you've probably had some type of imaging study that was instrumental in finding your liver tumor. Now your liver specialist may ask you to undergo further tests to try to pinpoint the exact nature of the tumor, to detect its exact location, and to determine whether or not it can be removed, or resected, easily.

A radiologist will view your imaging studies to determine the following:

- Is there one tumor, or are there many?
- Where is the tumor located?
- How big is it?
- What is the tumor's blood supply, or vascularity, like? Is the tumor encroaching, encasing, or invading the blood vessels in the liver?
- Are there features of liver scarring, or cirrhosis? One would suspect cirrhosis if the liver appeared small, shrunken, bumpy (nodular), and distorted. If you have cirrhosis, your spleen may be

enlarged, and there may be prominent veins around both of these organs.

- Are there any other clues as to the nature of the mass? For example, a star-shaped scar in the middle of a lesion is characteristic of both a benign liver tumor called focal nodular hyperplasia (FNH) and a rare malignant tumor known as fibrolamellar hepatoma.

These are the types of scans that you may need to have so that the radiologist can address these questions:

- **Ultrasound.** During an ultrasound test, high-frequency sound waves are directed toward the body. When these waves bounce back, their "echoes" are used to produce images of the internal organs. Before this painless and radiation-free procedure to view your liver, the technician will apply a lubricant gel to your abdomen. He or she then will move a device called a transducer over your abdomen, and the images that this device transmits will be shown on a video screen.

- **CAT scan.** This test is used to view the liver and its surrounding organs. Sometimes a special CAT scan called a CAT angiogram can be done to look at the arteries and veins within the liver. CAT is a painless X-ray technique that creates three-dimensional images of the body's internal structures. These images, which reflect the density of organs and tumors, are presented as cross-sections, or "slices," of the part of the body being scanned. CAT angiography sometimes involves the injection of a contrast dye that travels to the tumor. The scan then will show the tumor and its blood supply very clearly. Generally a CAT is taken while you are lying on a bed or table, and the technician moves the X-ray machine around you.

- **Magnetic resonance imaging (MRI) or magnetic resonance angiography (MRA).** MRI is similar to CAT in that it creates "sectional" images of the body. However, with MRI a magnet and a radio signal, rather than radiation, are used to produce these images. Like the other imaging techniques that I have described, MRI is painless, although some patients feel quite claustrophobic, because the scan is performed while the person is lying inside a large, tubelike machine.

- **Technetium sulfur colloid liver scan (liver-spleen scan).** The liver-spleen scan uses very small amounts of radioactive tracers to look at the liver and spleen. You will be given, intravenously, an isotope called technetium. This is perfectly safe. Once technetium is taken up by your liver, you will be asked to lie on a table, and the activity of the radiation that is emitted from your liver will be recorded by an imaging device. I sometimes order this type of scan if I'm trying to determine whether we're dealing with focal nodular hyperplasia.

We try not to do any unnecessary tests, but sometimes a number of tests are needed. I tell my patients that we'll do these scans in a certain logical sequence. Sometimes the first or second test may give us pretty definitive information so that we're confident of what we're dealing with, but sometimes, unfortunately, after all of these tests the true nature of the liver lesion is still not clear.

BIOPSY

What is the role of the liver biopsy in the diagnosis of liver tumors? If the radiologist finds a single lesion, and there is concern that it's a hepatoma arising within the liver (not a tumor that has appeared because of cancer elsewhere in the body), I usually don't recommend a biopsy. This procedure, which involves removing a small piece of the tumor for examination under the microscope, may be risky because bleeding can occur with benign as well as malignant tumors (many of which are very vascular, which means that they have a rich blood supply). A biopsy also may be risky because on rare occasions, with malignant tumors, the procedure itself can disperse cancerous cells along the tract where the needle was inserted. This "tumor seeding" may cause the cancer to spread. Finally, the amount of tissue retrieved may not be sufficient to make a diagnosis anyway. I don't feel that it's worthwhile to go through this risk if, in the end, we're no better off than we were before.

We do perform a biopsy if there are several lesions and we're pretty sure that they represent metastatic disease (for example, the patient has breast cancer or colon cancer). In this case, the cancer already has spread, so tumor seeding is not an issue. If the tumors are metastatic and they don't appear to have a very rich blood supply, a radiologist can do a "directed biopsy"; that is, he or she can use an ultrasound probe or CAT scan to pinpoint the exact location of the tumors in the liver and direct the biopsy needle into one of the metastatic lesions, thus ensuring procurement of a good specimen.

The biopsy procedure is described in more detail in chapter 2.

AFTER THE DIAGNOSIS, WHAT HAPPENS NEXT?

Once you've been through this diagnostic workup, your liver specialist probably can attach a name to the tumor that has worried you and your family since it was first discovered. Next you'll want to know how this sort of tumor behaves and what can be done about it.

Let's talk a little bit about the various types of benign and malignant liver tumors and the different treatment options. There are many types of treatment, depending upon the type of tumor you have. Your overall health, the condition of your liver, and the number of your tumors and where they are located are all important factors in determining which is best for you.

BENIGN TUMORS OF THE LIVER

The three major common benign tumors of the liver are called hepatic hemangioma, hepatic adenoma, and focal nodular hyperplasia.

HEPATIC HEMANGIOMA

Hepatic hemangiomas are so common that they may be found in up to 7 percent of all people at autopsy. If you've been diagnosed with this type of tumor, you may wonder what it looks like. Most (90 percent) are single lesions located on the right lobe of the liver. These lesions range in size from a few millimeters to 25 centimeters. A hemangioma is a tumor made up of cells that form blood vessels, so an abnormal collection or cluster of blood vessels may be present too.

SYMPTOMS. Most often, a hepatic hemangioma causes no symptoms, but sometimes there may be bleeding within the tumor or (rarely) a blood clot that may cause pain.

DIAGNOSIS. These tumors can be identified through ultrasound, CT, and MRI. Because a hepatic hemangioma can bleed if a needle is inserted into it, if your liver specialist thinks that you have this type of tumor, he or she won't do a liver biopsy.

TREATMENT. Although being diagnosed with a tumor is traumatic in and of itself, if you have no symptoms and your doctor is pretty confident that the tumor is a hepatic hemangioma, you should consider yourself very fortunate. Very often, no treatment for these benign tumors is necessary. Your liver specialist may repeat an imaging study, such as an ultrasound, six months after the initial diagnosis to make sure that nothing has changed, and then that's pretty much the end of the workup—no further screening is called for.

In the rare circumstance that you have pain or that, despite doing imaging studies, your liver specialist and radiologist are unable to determine with confidence what kind of tumor you have, you may be referred to a surgeon who can remove it, because you wouldn't want to take the chance that it's malignant.

HEPATIC ADENOMA

Another type of benign tumor of the liver, hepatic adenoma, is most common in adults, especially in women in their reproductive years. One risk factor for this type of lesion is the use of birth control pills for five years or more. Up to 90 percent of patients with hepatic adenomas have taken them, and the risk of developing this tumor increases the longer these contraceptives are used. Other risk factors for this tumor include:

- **Diabetes**
- **Glycogen storage disease,** a rare metabolic disease that affects the body's ability to break down blood sugar
- **Tyrosinemia,** an inherited condition in which there is abnormal metabolism of an amino acid called tyrosine

These tumors are very vascular; that is, they have a rich blood supply. They usually appear as solitary masses bigger than 10 centimeters. In spite of their size, however, hepatic adenomas rarely become malignant, and the prognosis for women who have been diagnosed with these tumors is usually very good.

SYMPTOMS. If you have a hepatic adenoma, you may have no symptoms and your physician may have discovered this benign tumor by chance while doing a radiologic scan for another reason. One-half to one-third of patients with a hepatic adenoma have abdominal pain, though. Rarely, this tumor can rupture and bleed into the abdominal cavity. When this happens, patients may experience severe abdominal pain, feel weak, or even faint because of enormous blood loss. This is a medical emergency that requires surgery to control the bleeding and remove the tumor.

DIAGNOSIS. Laboratory blood test results may be normal, although some patients have a low red blood cell count (anemia). Liver function tests (LFTs; see pages 74–77) may be normal or mildly elevated. With this type of tumor, the tumor marker known as alpha-fetoprotein (AFP) is normal. Radiologic studies such as CAT, MRI, or angiography may show features suggesting that the liver tumor is an adenoma. Because of the risk of bleeding, a percutaneous needle liver biopsy should not be done.

TREATMENT. I recommend that women with a diagnosis of hepatic adenoma stop taking oral contraceptives. Sometimes, the tumor may regress when birth control pills are stopped. If it doesn't disappear or if the patient was not taking birth control pills, surgical removal of the tumor usually is called for because of the risk of bleeding and the rare transformation of these benign masses to malignant cancers. Surgery also may be necessary if there is diagnostic uncertainty as to whether the mass is a hepatic adenoma or another kind of tumor.

FOCAL NODULAR HYPERPLASIA

Unlike hepatic adenoma, another benign tumor called focal nodular hyperplasia (FNH) has no malignant potential whatsoever, so the prognosis for patients with these types of tumors is usually excellent.

We don't know what causes these rare masses. They usually appear as a single lesion that may be either small or large. These tumors don't rupture, and bleeding is very uncommon. As with hepatic adenomas, FNH is most common in women of childbearing age. However, there is no proven relationship between the development of this tumor and the use of oral contraceptives. Children, older women, and men can develop this tumor, too.

SYMPTOMS. If you have FNH, you probably will not have symptoms, although you could have some pain on your right side, beneath your rib cage (where your liver is located).

DIAGNOSIS. Blood test results generally provide no clues as to this diagnosis. On CAT or MRI scans, however, a radiologist often will see a star-shaped scar in the middle of this tumor. Although this sign can appear with other tumors, this characteristic scar in a patient who has no symptoms and no positive tumor markers on blood tests is highly suggestive of FNH. A liver-spleen (technetium sulfur colloid scan) also can be useful in diagnosing this tumor.

One of my patients was a forty-three-year-old architect who was referred to me by her primary care physician after a liver mass was found on an ultrasound scan. This imaging scan was performed because she had experienced vague abdominal discomfort and bloating, and her doctor suspected that she may have a gallstone problem.

When she came to my office, I took a detailed medical history, and she told me that she had taken birth control pills for a couple of years several years ago. She was taking no other medications, and she didn't have any risk factors for viral hepatitis. Furthermore, she had no family history of liver cancer, and she hadn't lost weight. All of these details were reassuring: it seemed unlikely that she had a malignant tumor.

I ordered some special blood tests to look for tumor markers and to test for markers of viral hepatitis, and the results were normal. Then I obtained a CAT scan, which showed a 4-cm lesion on the right lobe of her liver. This lesion, which had a characteristic scar in the middle, appeared to be an FNH.

Although my patient was quite alarmed about having a liver tumor, I told her that given this constellation of findings, the tumor was probably benign, and a skilled liver surgeon would be able to remove it easily. She went off to Yellowstone for a vacation with her family, and while there she experienced an episode of mild pain on her right side. After she returned, she had another episode of pain. We decided to operate, not because we feared that the tumor might be malignant, but because it was causing significant discomfort in this person who led a very active life. There may have been bleeding within the tumor, or there may have been twisting on the "stalk" that attached this mass to the liver.

She had surgery, and the tumor was determined with certainty to be an FNH. That was five years ago, and she has done extremely well since then.

TREATMENT. In contrast to hepatic adenoma, for which surgery is recommended for most patients (since there is concern about the potential for development of a malignancy and because a significant number of these tumors can bleed and cause severe pain), in FNH patients surgery is indicated only in a minority of patients who develop symptoms. We also recommend surgery if we're not certain about the precise diagnosis despite extensive radiologic testing.

Thus, if you have no symptoms, your laboratory blood tests are reassuring, your liver-spleen scan is normal, and your doctors are confident that this tumor is truly an FNH, then no treatment is required. You'll simply need to see your physician periodically for an office visit.

MALIGNANT TUMORS OF THE LIVER

PRIMARY HEPATOCELLULAR CARCINOMA

Primary liver cancer, also called primary hepatocellular carcinoma or hepatoma, arises in the liver most often as a ball-like tumor that can spread to the tissue all around it. Hepatoma is one of the most common tumors in the world, and it causes from 500,000 to 1 million deaths globally each year.

INCIDENCE. The number of cases of hepatoma varies tremendously throughout the world as a result of different rates of exposure to the hepatitis B virus (HBV). In some areas of Asia (such as the People's Republic of China, Hong Kong, and Taiwan) and sub-Saharan Africa, for example, the incidence is extremely high. More than 50 percent of all cases of hepatoma occur in the People's Republic of China, where the annual incidence of hepatoma is 137,000 cases. In contrast, in the United States, this type of cancer represents less than 2.5 percent of all malignancies, although the incidence of hepatoma in this country appears to be rising.

In a recent study that examined the incidence of proven hepatoma over two periods (1976–1980 and 1991–1995), the mortality attributable to hepatoma was shown to have risen by about 40 percent. This study also showed a significant increase in the incidence of this type of tumor among forty- to sixty-year-olds, and noted that the highest incidence was among black men. The likely explanation is that there is a large pool of people with long-standing hepatitis C virus (HCV) infection in whom the disease has progressed to cirrhosis. I'm hopeful that in the not-too-distant future, we'll see less cases of hepatoma because of universal vaccination against HBV and because of widespread and effective treatment of chronic HCV with drugs like ribavirin and interferon.

Hepatoma is two to six times more common in men than in women. In the United States, it's most common in people in their fifties and sixties. Elsewhere, in areas where this cancer is quite prevalent, it tends to affect people who are younger than age forty.

RISK FACTORS. One in four patients with this type of cancer has no known risk factors. Others have had a disease or chronic viral infection, often for many years, that has led to liver scarring, or cirrhosis. When cirrhosis occurs, the liver cells die and regenerate in an unhealthy fashion, and they can become cancerous. In the United States, the two most common diseases associated with hepatoma—and the diseases that carry the worst prognosis—are alcoholic cirrhosis and chronic HCV infection.

My colleague, Dr. Keith Stuart, is a liver cancer expert at the Beth Israel Deaconess Cancer Center in Boston. He notes that a lot of patients with hepatoma are ex-alcoholics. "It's not fair," he says, "but you only seem to get this tumor if you quit drinking—otherwise you don't live long enough to get the tumor. It takes about twenty to thirty years to develop it. If you keep drinking, you die from acute problems." Fortunately, the incidence of alcoholic cirrhosis appears to be declining.

Other chronic liver diseases that have been associated with an increased risk of primary liver cancer are:

- **Idiopathic genetic hemochromatosis,** an iron overload disorder in which excessive amounts of iron are absorbed from the gastrointestinal tract and deposited elsewhere in the body, where they can cause diabetes, cirrhosis, and heart failure (see chapter 11).
- **Alpha$_1$antitrypsin deficiency,** a deficiency of a plasma protein that is produced in the liver. This deficiency may lead to cirrhosis and to emphysema (even in nonsmokers).
- **Hereditary tyrosinemia,** a disorder involving abnormal metabolism of an amino acid called tyrosine.

Finally, the development of hepatoma may be related to exposure to environmental toxins like aflatoxin (a mold that grows on certain grains and contaminates drinking water in some parts of Africa and Southeast Asia). Thorotrast (thorium dioxide), a radiologic contrast material that is no longer in use, also has been linked to the development of this type of cancer. Some studies have indicated that cigarette smoking may be a factor, too.

PROGNOSIS. Dr. Keith Stuart notes that hepatoma is different than other forms of cancer in that "people's survival is not based just on the size of the cancer or the aggressiveness of the lesion. With breast cancer or colon cancer, we want to know what the cancer is like and what it's doing. In this type of cancer we want to know what the cirrhosis is like. So many people [with this kind of tumor] have cirrhosis, and we've had many people in whom we've been able to control the tumor but they died of cirrhosis. So it's really a combination of what the tumor does and how bad the cirrhosis is that determines how long people live."

The average survival of patients with symptoms of hepatoma is six weeks to six months after diagnosis, but there are exceptions. Eleven years ago, Dr. Stuart diagnosed hepatoma in a nun who works as a missionary, and with treatment, she has done remarkably well.

SYMPTOMS. If you have hepatoma, you may have no symptoms other than those related to cirrhosis (such as loss of appetite, weakness, abdominal pain, and jaundice, or yellowing of the skin and the whites of the eyes). In addition to these symptoms, you may develop a fever, lose weight, and have watery diarrhea or bone pain. Patients with this type of cancer also can develop a swollen, fluid-filled abdomen that may make them look pregnant. This condition is called ascites. Other rare symptoms of hepatoma are severe flushing, weakness, headaches, and tremors.

DIAGNOSIS. Most of the time there are no clues to the presence of hepatoma. Your doctor may notice signs of cirrhosis (such as red palms and spider veins), and sometimes a painful lump can be felt over the liver. While listening to the sounds arising from the liver, the hepatologist also may hear an abnormal "bruit," a little hum caused by the increased blood flow of this very vascular tumor.

Blood tests. High concentrations of a protein called alpha-fetoprotein (AFP) are found in 70 percent of patients with hepatoma in the United States.

Radiologic tests. Ultrasounds, CAT scans, MRIs, and sometimes MRAs (magnetic resonance angiography scans) are useful for assessing the extent of the hepatoma and revealing the blood supply to it. On rare occasions, a nuclear medicine scan called a gallium scan is used to detect this type of tumor. Your liver specialist, working with an experienced radiologist, will determine which imaging study to do and how to interpret the results of these tests.

Biopsy. If you have hepatoma, your doctor may not perform a liver biopsy because of the risk of bleeding and possible spread of tumor cells.

TREATMENT. What are your treatment options if you have hepatoma? First let's look at traditional cancer therapies that are *not* used for hepatoma. Radiation is seldom used for liver tumors, because the liver may be very sensitive to radiation—more sensitive than the tumor is. The risk is that we may wind up causing something called radiation hepatitis and damaging the liver before we've actually destroyed the tumor.

Likewise, traditional chemotherapy—or highly toxic drugs administered to the whole body—generally aren't given, because the liver treats such toxins as it does all others: it tries to cleanse the body of them. In some cases, though, chemotherapy drugs are injected directly into the tumor. I'll describe this method shortly.

Treatment options that *are* used for hepatoma include:

1. Surgery to remove the liver tumor
2. A liver transplant
3. Chemoembolization
4. Alcohol ablation
5. Radiofrequency ablation
6. Hormone therapy
7. Potential new therapies

Now let's look more closely at these choices.

• **Surgery: partial hepatectomy** (removal of part of the liver). Surgery may well be the best treatment option, although it may not be possible if your liver function is severely impaired because of advanced cirrhosis, or if you have too many tumors or other serious medical problems. Unfortunately, most patients with hepatoma are not good candidates for surgical resection. The patients who have the best outcomes with surgery have small (less than 5 cm in diameter) and solitary tumors that are confined to the liver. The five-year survival rates after surgery range from 30 percent to as high as 90 percent.

Cryosurgery. Occasionally, if a tumor cannot be removed surgically, a surgeon may freeze it with supercold liquid nitrogen, and in the process, destroy it. This procedure is called cryosurgery.

• **Liver transplantation.** If you have a single, small (less than 5 cm) tumor, or three or less tumors that are smaller than 3 centimeters, you may be a candidate for a liver transplant, which involves removing the diseased liver, tumor and all, and replacing it with a new liver from a donor. If this major surgical operation is done, it should be performed early, before the tumor or tumors have a chance to grow.

Recent studies have shown survival rates of as high as 75 percent five years after a liver transplant for patients who had hepatoma. However, these patients had tumors that were smaller than 3 centimeters, had less than three tumors, and had no tumors that invaded the blood vessels within the liver. These encouraging results also were contingent upon a very short waiting time between the diagnosis of hepatoma and the actual liver transplant. As I'll explain in chapter 13, the waiting period for a donor liver may be a year or two, or even longer in some parts of the country. During this waiting time, the tumor can grow and disqualify a person for a liver transplant.

• **Embolization of the bleeding vessel.** Besides surgical removal, a hepatoma can be destroyed by choking or cutting off its blood supply (by injecting small particles into the blood vessels that feed it) or by administering toxic chemotherapy directly into the tumor. In a procedure called transarterial chemoembolization (TACE), the blood vessels that supply the tumor are blocked with gelfoam metal coils. High concentrations of chemotherapy drugs (sometimes in a solution that promotes their retention within the tumor) are then infused directly into the tumor.

TACE is used in patients who have large tumors that would not be suitable for other forms of treatment. Although a number of studies have shown that this type of treatment can lead to a reduction in tumor growth, this therapy is not associated with improvement in survival. At the hospital where I work, patients who undergo this procedure are selected carefully, and a number of factors, including the size of the tumor, the age of the patient, and whether or not he or she has alcoholic cirrhosis, are considered. Approximately 250 of our patients with hepatoma have been treated by this method over the last ten years. About 60 percent of the time, these tumors shrink. This procedure also appears to prolong people's lives—overall patients are living one to one and a half years longer than they would otherwise.

In spite of these gains, there are some downsides to chemotherapeutic embolization. As I mentioned earlier, one of the problems with using chemotherapy to treat primary liver cancers is that the liver treats this toxin just as it does others that it encounters—it tries to purge the body of it. So there are a lot of side effects, such as abdominal pain and fever. This response to treatment sometimes is referred to as postembolization syndrome.

Moreover, even though liver surgeons direct the catheter that carries the chemotherapeutic drug specifically at the tumor, the liver tissue surrounding the tumor may be damaged in the process. If you have cirrhosis, you may not have much liver to spare. Generally, then, this option is used for patients whose symptoms cannot be controlled by other means.

• **Injection of alcohol into the tumor (alcohol ablation).** Another way to kill and shrink tumors and improve one's chance for survival is to inject a solution containing 95 percent alcohol directly into the tumor. This therapy may need to be repeated several times.

In one study of more than 100 patients in whom this technique was used, the five-year survival rate was approximately 50 percent. These patients had Child's class A cirrhosis, the most mild form of cirrhosis (see chapter 9). The success of alcohol ablation is monitored with ultrasound or CAT. It's generally well tolerated. Complications such as liver or kidney failure or bleeding within the abdomen occur in less than 5 percent of cases. In some patients, this treatment causes abdominal pain.

I recommend alcohol ablation for patients who have a single 3- to 4-centimeter tumor, but not enough healthy liver tissue to safely withstand liver surgery.

- **Radiofrequency ablation.** For small tumors, radiofrequency ablation (RFA) is another treatment option. Ultrasound is used to locate the tumor, and then a needle is inserted into the tumor. Radio waves pass through the needle, generating heat and killing the tumor in the process.

- **Hormone therapies.** Drugs such as Tamoxifen, which has been used for patients with breast cancer, are under study for treatment of hepatomas, yet preliminary results have been disappointing. It's possible that future studies will show some potential benefit.

- **New and emerging therapies.** In a process called angiogenesis, tumors can form new blood vessels from existing ones. New drugs called angiostatin and endostatin someday may be used to block tumor growth by cutting off the blood supply that feeds them. Experiments in animals such as mice have shown that these drugs can shrink tumors and in some cases make them disappear. These drugs are being tested in people, and if they work, they could turn out to be extremely useful in managing hepatomas.

FIBROLAMELLAR HEPATOMA

Another malignant tumor that accounts for 1 to 2 percent of all liver tumors is called fibrolamellar hepatoma. This type of tumor affects both men and women equally. It's not related to chronic HBV or HCV infections or to the use of birth control pills. Most (90–95 percent) patients with this type of tumor *do not* have cirrhosis. Patient survival is better than that seen with patients with primary liver cancer (the usual form of hepatoma).

DIAGNOSIS. AFP levels are normal or mildly elevated in most patients with fibrolamellar hepatoma. Also, two blood tests can be elevated abnormally just with this type of tumor:

1. Serum unsaturated vitamin B_{12}-binding capacity
2. A hormone called plasma neurotensin

If these two tests are abnormal, that would signal the likelihood that this tumor is fibrolamellar hepatoma.

On a CAT scan, one may see a central scar with calcification of the tumor. This finding also may be associated with a benign tumor called focal nodular hyperplasia, which I discussed earlier.

TREATMENT. Surgery is recommended for patients with this type of tumor more often than for patients who have the usual form of hepatoma. Patients who do not have cirrhosis (liver scarring) have a better outcome. For some patients, liver transplantation is an option.

CANCER THAT SPREADS TO THE LIVER

The liver is a large organ that has a rich blood supply, so cancer commonly spreads, or metastasizes, to it from the colon, pancreas, gallbladder, stomach, lung, breast, ovaries, testes, and skin (melanoma). Malignant tumors that metastasize to the liver less frequently are thyroid and prostate tumors.

SYMPTOMS

If you have metastatic lesions to the liver, you may have no symptoms, or you may have nonspecific symptoms such as fatigue, lack of appetite, abdominal discomfort, or ascites. Occasionally patients also have jaundice. One of the striking things about metastatic cancer is that jaundice, which develops because of replacement of liver tissue by the tumor, is a very late finding.

Sometimes jaundice is due not to a tumor but to other factors such as a large lymph node that compresses the bile ducts coming out of the liver. In this case, jaundice is not a late event. A malignant tumor called lymphoma in the neck or chest (such as Hodgkin's disease) also may cause deep jaundice even though there is no tumor metastasis to the liver. If the tumor responds to chemotherapy, the jaundice may resolve.

DIAGNOSIS

To look for metastasis to the liver, laboratory blood tests are routinely done. Liver-spleen scans will reveal lesions that are larger than 2 centimeters in diameter, and ultrasound and CAT scans may show smaller lesions.

A liver biopsy may be necessary to confirm the findings of the imaging study or studies. Usually this biopsy is done by a radiologist who directs a needle into the tumor using ultrasound guidance.

TREATMENT

The treatment for patients with metastatic disease to the liver is best carried out by an oncologist. Sometimes these tumors respond well to chemotherapy.

SUMMARY

In summary, tumors of the liver are not always malignant, or cancerous. Indeed, one of the most common tumors in the liver is a benign mass called a hemangioma. Even if a tumor is malignant, it often can be removed by a surgical procedure known as a hepatectomy or destroyed with various forms of local treatment. These forms of treatment can be well tolerated and result in striking success.

Intense research is being carried out to understand the causes of liver tumors and find better tests and treatments for them. Undoubtedly, we will make promising advances in the years to come.

The incidence of cancer of the liver (a major cause of which is chronic HBV infection) should decrease dramatically with implementation of childhood HBV vaccination. The Global Alliance for Vaccines and Immunizations was founded in 1999 by the World Health Organization, UNICEF, and the World Bank. It recently received a donation of $150 million from the Bill and Melinda Gates Foundation. What a wonderful gift!

13

Liver Transplants

We met in New York City. Philip was working in a restaurant near the hospital where my mother was fighting cancer, and after visiting her, I'd stop there for a burger on the way home.

I had a crush on him, maybe because he comes from a great big Italian family and he's a great storyteller.

Anyway, one night he did not ask—he said that we were going to go to dinner. And we haven't been apart since.

—Karen Scolaro

If the liver is the seat of the soul, then Karen and Philip Scolaro are the ultimate soulmates. That's because on December 10, 1998, liver transplant surgeons at the hospital where I work, Boston's Beth Israel Deaconess Medical Center, removed more than half of Philip's liver and implanted it into his wife, Karen, after her own diseased liver had been removed.

In the future, this new procedure, which is called living-donor liver transplantation, most likely will be used more and more instead of traditional liver transplant procedures, which require the use of a liver from a person who has died. The growing interest in living donation stems from the severe shortage of donor organs just as the demand for livers is skyrocketing. This great escalation in the need for livers is due, in part, to the "silent epidemic" of hepatitis C, the number-one reason for liver transplants in adults in the United States. A number of investigators have concluded that this epidemic will lead to a sixfold increase in the need for liver transplant procedures by the year 2008. Even in 1998, when 4,413 liver transplants were performed in this country, 12,070 patients with advanced liver disease were waiting for livers and 1,317 died while on the waiting list.

In this chapter, I'll tell you about how both living-donor and traditional ("cadaveric") transplant procedures came about, how the organ allocation system works in the United States today, and finally, and most importantly, what you can expect if your doctor recommends that you undergo a liver transplant because of end-stage chronic liver disease.

SOME BACKGROUND

Researchers first began experimenting with liver transplants in animals in the 1950s and 1960s.

In March 1963, at the University of Colorado in Denver, Dr. Thomas E. Starzl performed the first such procedure in a person. Unfortunately, this operation failed. Indeed, a number of subsequent attempts by his team and by surgeons in Boston and Paris were likewise unsuccessful.

One reason for these repeated failures early on was that the immune system of a transplant recipient tries to fight off the new organ as if it were a foreign invader. In 1966, however, a powerful new drug called antilymphocyte serum (ALS) became available in clinical protocols. This agent and other "immunosuppressant" drugs that were developed thereafter contributed greatly to the future success of liver transplant procedures, because they helped to check this immune response.

In spite of his initially disappointing results, Dr. Starzl went back to the laboratory and diligently continued his endeavors. And his dedication paid off: in July 1967, he performed what I believe to be one of the major medical achievements of the latter half of the twentieth century—the first successful liver transplant. This patient, a little girl who had a type of liver cancer called primary hepatocellular carcinoma, or hepatoma, lived for thirteen months after this operation before succumbing to recurrent cancer.

As the first liver transplants in humans were performed, many of the major obstacles to successful transplant operations that we think of today were not known or were only beginning to be considered. We weren't yet struggling to procure enough livers for transplantation; trying to determine which patients would receive donated livers; wrestling with legal definitions of brain death; or refining technically demanding aspects of the transplant operation. Over the last three decades, considerable worldwide experience has led to dramatic progress in these and many other areas. In the late 1970s, for instance, two more very effective immunosuppressants—cyclosporine and monoclonal antibodies—were developed. At the same time, scientists were making great strides in finding better ways to preserve donor organs.

Finally, in 1983, liver transplants moved from the experimental arena to become commonly accepted treatments for patients with severe liver disease. A major impetus for this change, and for the creation of many transplant centers in the United States, was a National Institutes of Health (NIH) consensus conference. This conference validated the clinical use of liver transplants and hailed these procedures as a "therapeutic modality for end-stage liver disease that deserves broader application." At that time, only two hospitals in the United States were performing liver transplants. Less than two decades later, there are more than 120 transplant centers. Even better, today survival rates after traditional liver transplants have risen to 85 percent one year after surgery and 70 percent three years after surgery.

ORGAN ALLOCATION

One year after the NIH consensus conference, Congress passed the National Organ Transplant Act (NOTA), which made the sale of human organs illegal and led to the creation of a national system for organ sharing. Since then, this system has been overseen by the United Network for Organ Sharing (UNOS), based in Richmond, Virginia. UNOS has a contract with the federal government to manage both transplant data and the allocation of livers.

The UNOS network, which is staffed every hour of the day and week, coordinates liver donation through a vast system of organ banks and transplant centers. UNOS maintains a central, computerized registry of all patients on the transplant waiting list, and it generates a list of potential candidates for each new organ that becomes available. This list depends on the liver's size and blood and tissue type, as well as on the severity of the recipient's liver disease and the length of time that she has been waiting for a liver.

Patients on the UNOS waiting list who live in the area where a donor organ becomes available are first in line to receive the liver. If none of the patients in that local area are a good match for the donor organ, it next becomes available to patients on the UNOS list in the broader region. (The system is organized into eleven regions throughout the country.) Finally, if no match is made within the donor's region, the liver becomes available to patients nationwide.

Although liver transplants usually aren't performed for patients who are over the age of seventy, age, gender, and race are not determining factors in who receives the few livers that are available. Furthermore, despite misperceptions to the contrary, livers are *not* distributed first to celebrities or to individuals who can pay the most for them. Confusion about this issue was fueled in 1995 when the baseball hero Mickey Mantle received a liver transplant just one day after he was listed with UNOS as having end-stage liver disease. However, his wait actually was not unusual for a patient with his medical condition in his area (Dallas) at that time. According to Dr. Maureen Martin, chief of the division of liver surgery and transplantation at Boston's Beth Israel Deaconess Medical Center, Mickey Mantle was the most seriously ill of the patients on the list in that area.

Recently, a movement has been underway to make distribution of organs need-based rather than location-based. In 1998 Arthur Caplan, a bioethicist at the University of Pennsylvania, wrote in the *New England Journal of Medicine* that "patients' chances of living or dying are shaped more by where they live than by how urgently they need a transplant." Donna Shalala, the U.S. Health and Human Services secretary, agrees, and she has proposed new guidelines to give livers to the sickest patients first, regardless of where they live. She sent a letter to members of Congress that said, "The National Organ Transplant Act of 1984 (NOTA) . . . was passed to create a national system in which an adequate supply of organs would be available on an equitable basis to patients throughout the nation. On both counts—the adequacy of organ supply as well as the equity in distribution—I believe we are falling short of the law's expectations. . . . In the worst case, patients die in areas where waiting times are long, while at the same time organs are being made available to less ill patients in areas with shorter waiting times."

Individuals who disagree with her proposal have expressed concerns about the costs involved in transporting livers over great distances, as well as the risk of damage to the organ that might occur while in transit. Some also have argued that it's not fair to give these scarce organs to the most gravely ill patients, who they believe may have less successful outcomes than patients who are healthier.

The National Academy of Science's Institute of Medicine is studying this issue. As of this writing, the location-based system is still in place.

ORGAN DONATION

Because of the extreme shortage of donors, efforts are being made around the country to educate the public about the growing need for organs. The Uniform Anatomical Gift Act says that anyone who is eighteen years or older can request that his organs be donated after death. If a child under the age of eighteen dies, his parents or legal guardians can donate that child's organs. Removal of the liver from a deceased person does not cost the donor's family anything. The American Liver Foundation, the American Kidney Foundation, and local organ procurement agencies all provide donor cards. In Massachusetts and most other states, the Registry of Motor Vehicles also has a place for donor information on driver's licenses.

> *My liver disease held me back from doing the things that I wanted to do. Now that I've had my transplant, I feel that I can finally start my life.*
>
> *You know, before [the transplant] I never thought much about donating organs, but now 90 percent of my friends have those stickers on their driver's licenses.*
> —SCOTT JACKLE, transplant recipient

If you are an organ donor, I want to assure you that your donation status *will not* affect your health care; that is, your doctors and nurses will still take all measures to save your life, and your liver will be removed only after brain death—a complete and irreversible absence of all brain function—has been declared legally. The team of doctors who remove the liver is totally separate from the team of doctors who treat the patient who eventually becomes the liver donor. In fact, the transplant team is not even notified about the liver until the donor's family has agreed to the donation. Moreover, to prevent any coercion of the donor, doctors have no idea who the recipient of the liver will be when they interview a potential donor (or, if the donor is deceased, his or her family).

Finally, Dr. Maureen Martin notes that removal of the liver for donation does not cause disfigurement of the body or a delay in transferring the body to a funeral home.

ORGAN QUALITY

If you are waiting for a liver transplant, you may be wondering about how healthy your "new" liver may be. A donor's liver may not be used if he had cancer or was infected with the human immunodeficiency virus (HIV) or hepatitis C virus (HCV), or if he had a bacterial or fungal infection. A donor's age generally is not relevant, though. Recent studies have shown that livers from donors who are over the age of sixty-five are not associated with a higher rate of complications or death in the organ recipient.

DO YOU NEED A LIVER TRANSPLANT?

Karen and Philip Scolaro had been married for three years, and she had been sick since shortly after their wedding with various symptoms of severe liver scarring, or cirrhosis. Off and on she struggled with a flu-like illness that robbed her of appetite. "We were trying desperately to get to the honeymoon," Karen says today, "but because I kept getting sick, we never got there."

It was the end of 1996, and Karen, who had been diagnosed with severe liver disease a year earlier, went into free fall. She almost died when varices, engorged veins in her esophagus caused by the cirrhosis, "blew." When she woke up in the hospital five days later, she was told that she had lost so much blood that she had nearly died. By this point, her liver was so damaged by cirrhosis that it was no longer purging her blood of toxins like ammonia, which is formed in the simple process of digesting food. As such poisons accumulated in her body, they affected her mind and made her sleepy and disoriented. The only way to keep this mental confusion (called hepatic encephalopathy) at bay was to consume lactulose, a syrupy medicine, several times each day.

Then, in early 1997, a parachute of sorts opened. Karen's gastroenterologist in New Hampshire sent a letter to my colleague, Dr. Fredric Gordon, who then was the medical director of liver transplantation at Boston's Beth Israel Deaconess Medical Center.

Shortly thereafter, Karen and Philip Scolaro drove to Boston and met with this liver doctor, whose notes from the office visit that day concluded, "Ms. Scolaro is a very reasonable candidate for liver transplantation."

CONDITIONS FOR WHICH TRANSPLANTS MAY BE REQUIRED

CIRRHOSIS DUE TO CHRONIC HEPATITIS INFECTION OR ALCOHOL. Your physician may recommend that you undergo a liver transplant procedure if, like Karen, you have end-stage liver disease because of liver scarring (cirrhosis) with potential or actual life-threatening complications. Advanced cirrhosis may be caused by chronic HBV or chronic HCV infection, alcoholic liver disease, and a number of other illnesses.

PRIMARY BILIARY CIRRHOSIS (PBC) AND PRIMARY SCLEROSING CHOLANGITIS (PSC). Liver diseases marked by blockage of bile flow, such as primary biliary cirrhosis (see chapter 10) and primary sclerosing cholangitis (see page 159), also can lead to cirrhosis and complications that may necessitate a liver transplant.

In patients with PBC, this operation may improve survival (one-year survival is as high as 95 percent, and five-year survival is approximately 80 percent). It also may relieve symptoms such as severe and protracted itching that cannot be controlled by any other method, as well as symptoms of end-stage liver disease, such as disabling encephalopathy and bleeding from esophageal varices.

Transplantation also may be helpful for patients with PBC who develop severe osteoporosis with fractures, although it may take twelve to eighteen months after the transplant before improvement is seen.

INBORN METABOLIC DISORDERS. Hemochromatosis, a disorder involving deposits of excess amounts of iron in the body, and Wilson's disease, a disorder involving excessive deposits of copper in the body, can cause cirrhosis that is so severe that a liver transplant may be called for.

LIVER TUMORS. Liver transplantation also is an option for people who cannot undergo surgical removal of a benign or malignant tumor because of its location or because of severe underlying liver disease (see chapter 13). The three-year survival rate for patients who have received liver transplants because of a malignant tumor called hepatoma is less than 50 percent. However, survival is as good as 90 percent for patients with a single tumor that is less than 5 centimeters in diameter or patients with three or fewer tumors that are 3 centimeters or smaller in diameter.

ACUTE FULMINANT LIVER FAILURE. Liver transplantation is also an approved option for patients who suddenly become severely ill with a condition called acute fulminant liver failure, or severe liver dysfunction that comes on swiftly and can rapidly lead to hepatic encephalopathy, which is characterized by the type of mental confusion that Karen experienced. Untreated, this condition can lead to coma, but if a patient with acute liver failure is referred immediately to a transplant center and if a donor is found in time, the survival rate can be 70 to 80 percent. Many of these patients are younger than age forty and do not have coexisting health problems, so they often do very well with a transplant.

SEVERE LIVER DISEASES IN CHILDREN. A child may need to have a liver transplant if he or she has any of the following disorders that has led to severe liver damage:

- Biliary atresia, a condition in which damage to the bile ducts leads to scarring, or cirrhosis

- Alagille's syndrome, a disease caused by blockage of bile flow in the liver
- Chronic hepatitis B or C viral infections
- Fulminant liver failure
- Certain benign and malignant tumors of the liver

If you or your child has one of the disorders that I've just described, how will you know if and when you'll need a liver transplant? Your physician may refer you for a liver transplant if you have one or more complications; if there is evidence that your liver disease is getting worse; or if you have fulminant liver failure.

The kinds of complications that may signal deterioration of your condition include:

- Fluid buildup in the abdomen (ascites)
- Infection of the ascitic fluid (spontaneous bacterial peritonitis)
- Variceal bleeding, or bleeding from engorged veins in the esophagus
- Mental confusion or coma due to hepatic encephalopathy
- A severe and persistent blood-clotting disorder (coagulopathy) because the liver is no longer producing blood-clotting factors properly
- A severe metabolic bone disease (hepatic osteodystrophy)
- Severe malnutrition
- Certain malignant tumors in the liver (see chapter 13)

Your liver specialist also may recommend a liver transplant if tests of liver function indicate that your liver condition has worsened considerably. You may, for instance, develop:

- Jaundice, or yellowing of the skin and the whites of the eyes, after you have had stable cirrhosis. If this occurs, a blood test that measures a bile pigment called bilirubin will reveal a bilirubin level that is higher than 3.0 mg/dl.
- An abnormally low level of the protein called albumin in your blood (this condition is called hypoalbuminemia); your physician will diagnose significant hypoalbuminemia if a blood test shows that you have a serum albumin level that is less than 3.0 g/dl.

- A blood-clotting disorder (coagulopathy); in this case, a blood test called prothrombin time will be more than 3 seconds greater than normal.

CONTRAINDICATIONS FOR A LIVER TRANSPLANT

Now that you know why a liver transplant may be called for, let's talk about factors that may prevent you from having this operation. In medical jargon, these factors are called contraindications.

ABSOLUTE CONTRAINDICATIONS

Absolute contraindications are factors that would prohibit a liver transplant because the outcome of this procedure most likely would be extremely poor. These factors include

- Uncontrolled infection outside the liver (such as HIV infection or blood infection)
- Malignancies outside the liver other than certain skin cancers such as squamous cell and basal cell carcinoma
- Severe heart or lung disease
- Current alcohol or drug abuse
- Insufficient family or social support

RELATIVE CONTRAINDICATIONS

The second type of contraindications, relative contraindications, may lead to a higher risk of death and disease after transplant, but in exceptional situations, this procedure may be carried out. These factors include

- Advanced age (over age seventy)
- A blood clot in the portal vein, which carries blood from the intestines to the liver. This type of clot occurs in 15 percent of patients with cirrhosis
- Severe kidney disease

- Severe liver cancer (primary hepatocellular carcinoma, or hepatoma), or a liver tumor that is larger than 5 centimeters (see chapter 13)
- Advanced malnutrition

WHEN YOUR DOCTOR RECOMMENDS A LIVER TRANSPLANT

If you have no contraindications and your gastroenterologist or hepatologist recommends a liver transplant to treat your end-stage liver disease, these are the steps that lie ahead of you:

1. You will be evaluated by the transplant team at a medical center where liver transplants are performed.
2. If the transplant team determines that you are an acceptable candidate for a liver transplant, they will register you on the UNOS waiting list.
3. You will wait!
4. If a donor organ becomes available, your transplant team will be notified, and they will decide whether or not to accept the new organ.
5. If the organ is accepted and you are in good condition for major surgery, you will have your operation.
6. You will go through a recovery period and will take lifelong immunosuppressant drug therapy.

EVALUATION BY THE TRANSPLANT TEAM

Karen Scolaro's liver transplant evaluation was a three-day outpatient "crash course" during which she learned about what a transplant would entail, how much it would cost, and what she could expect in terms of drug therapy and recovery afterward. She asked a lot of questions.

Between her meetings with a transplant nurse, a social worker, an infectious disease specialist, a dietitian, a psychiatrist, and a financial counselor, she was tapped for blood, scanned, and scanned some more. And her new doctors asked her a lot of questions, too.

THE TRANSPLANT TEAM

The evaluation is a good opportunity to become more acquainted with the transplant team, whose skill and guidance will be essential in the coming days. There may be a core team that is composed of a hepatologist, a transplant surgeon, and an anesthesiologist.

Ancillary members, who also will be involved intimately in your care, may include:

- **A transplant nurse coordinator,** who will go over what you can expect in terms of waiting period, medications after transplant, and so forth.
- **A psychiatrist or psychologist,** who can talk with you about chemical dependency issues, your fears and concerns, and the impact of this major operation on your family.
- **A social worker,** who also can guide you and your family through this major event.
- **A nutritionist,** who can give you advice about your diet both before and after the transplant.
- **An infectious disease consultant,** who will make sure that when your immune system is suppressed, an infection that has been dormant, or "subclinical," isn't activated.
- **A financial counselor,** who can help you sort out what your insurance will cover. As of this writing, traditional cadaveric transplants can cost up to $500,000 for the transplant and treatment in the first year after surgery (this includes $20,000 to acquire the liver from the organ bank). Living donation is somewhat less expensive than traditional liver transplants.

  Each insurance plan is different. Sometimes insurance companies will pay for the procedure but not the antirejection medicines that must be taken afterward. Since monthly bills for immunosuppressants can exceed $3,000 per month, some pharmaceutical companies have free care plans to supply immunosuppressant drugs to patients who would not be able to afford them otherwise.

THE MEDICAL TESTS

In addition to your meetings with this group of specialists, you probably will be asked to go through a series of diagnostic tests to assess the severity of your disease and look for any complications and coexisting conditions that you may have.

You may meet with one or more physicians to go through your medical history, physical examination, and laboratory blood tests. Your transplant team also will want to assess your vital organs before you undergo the stress of surgery. This assessment may involve the following tests:

- Electrocardiogram (EKG) to make sure that you don't have a heart condition. A coronary arteriogram also may be done if you are at risk for coronary artery disease.
- Chest X-ray and pulmonary function tests to check your lungs.
- Twenty-four-hour urine collection to check your kidney function.
- Ultrasound, magnetic resonance imaging (MRI), or computed axial tomographic (CAT) scans of your liver to look for potential blockages and to determine your exact liver size.

THE OPTIONS

Dr. Elizabeth Pomfret, a transplant surgeon, notes that the option of a living donor transplant is usually presented when patients have their initial meeting with the evaluation team. A patient already may have heard of this procedure and may inform the transplant team that she has a relative who has offered to donate part of his liver. According to Dr. Pomfret, the surgeons also "target people who we think would be good candidates for living donation." For living donation, the patient has to have:

- A donor who is genetically or emotionally related, either a blood relative, a spouse or partner, or a very close friend.
- A donor with a compatible blood type, either the same blood type or type O blood, which is compatible with all blood types.

- A donor with a compatible liver size—the donor must have a liver that is at least as big as the recipient's, and preferably bigger. A tall, large man would be a suitable donor for a shorter, smaller woman, for instance, but not vice versa.

I'll tell you more about this newer transplant procedure later in this chapter.

GETTING ACCEPTED
INTO A TRANSPLANT PROGRAM

Every week at our medical center, the transplant team has a screening committee meeting. The cases of two to five patients, on average, are presented to the group. The team decides on the suitability of the candidate for transplantation based on her health status and social support. She may be accepted pending further workup and testing.

If you are approved for a transplant, your name, social security number, blood type, and ID number will be registered with the national centralized computer network overseen by UNOS. Your transplant team will also designate your case with a status number according to very specific information. They will use a uniform scoring system that's based on points for certain lab values and clinical signs. The three laboratory values that count are

- **Albumin,** which reflects how well your liver is synthesizing protein;
- **Prothrombin time,** which indicates how well your liver is producing blood clotting factors; and
- **Bilirubin,** which denotes how well your liver is handling this bile pigment.

In addition to these laboratory values, your UNOS status is based on the presence and degree of two clinical signs:

- **Ascites,** or fluid in the abdomen, and
- **Hepatic encephalopathy,** or the level of confusion that you may be experiencing because of the effect of liver failure on your brain.

Once your transplant team has counted up points based upon these objective factors, your case will be designated with a UNOS status number:

- *Status 1* is assigned to patients who are the most ill and may not survive more than a week without a new liver (for example, with fulminant liver failure caused by an acute viral infection). Such patients generally receive a liver transplant within a few days.
- *Status 2A* is given on an "interim" basis for patients who are in a critical care unit of a hospital and also have a life expectancy of less than one week.
- *Status 2B* is the designation for patients who have later stages of chronic liver disease and perhaps some of the signs of end-stage liver disease: persistent bleeding from veins in the esophagus (esophageal varices) despite treatment; severe kidney disease; a swollen, fluid-filled abdomen (ascites); "hepatohydrothorax," a large, often massive accumulation of fluid in the lining around the lung (the pleura) that is not responsive to treatment; or severe mental confusion (encephalopathy).
- *Status 3* is assigned to patients who are the least ill.
- *Status 4* is for "temporarily inactive" cases. This means that the patient went through the evaluation process and was referred to UNOS to be listed as needing a liver, but her status then improved. She may not need a liver at this time, but may need one in the future.

THE WAIT

Waiting for a donor liver was a huge emotional roller coaster.
The beeper would go off by accident, and we'd look at each other.
The first time it went off, we were sitting down having dinner. He
looked at me and said, "I've got this feeling this could be it."
—KAREN SCOLARO

In the United States, most patients wait six months to one year or longer for a donor liver; in some areas, the wait may be as long as two to three years. During this time, you will have regular appointments with both your local gastroenterologist and the physicians at the transplant center. They will examine you, run laboratory blood tests, and have you undergo ultrasound tests periodically. How can you cope with this wait? Many of my patients find that staying active and continuing their usual activities helps.

Karen Scolaro was on the UNOS waiting list for a cadaveric liver for two and a half years before she eventually underwent a living donor transplant. During her waiting period, she found that massage and swimming twice a week were helpful. She also tried to maintain some sense of humor. "I was all jaundiced," she recalls, "so I lit up the pool with my bright yellow eyes." Another transplant recipient, Scott Jackle, owns a bakery, and he continued to work from eight to fifteen hours a day right up until surgery. He says, "Working kept me going mentally. It gave me something to do." Counseling with a good therapist or social worker can also be beneficial at this time. Some patients attend transplant support groups that are run by the American Liver Foundation.

Finally, this is a time to garner the support of your family and friends. "This is the worst time in people's lives," Karen Scolaro says. "Not just their lives but the entire family's. If the family is not united in getting this accomplished, it's really not going to work. You really all have to say, 'Okay, this is what we've got to do.'"

Scott Jackle's family kept his bakery and twenty-five employees going through the holiday season while he was recuperating from his surgery. His girlfriend took off two and a half months from work to take care of him.

A LIVER BECOMES AVAILABLE

THE TRANSPLANT TEAM MAKES A DECISION

Dr. Pomfret explains that when one of her patients is "up next" on the UNOS list, she and the other transplant surgeons on the team may receive a call that there is, for example, a sixteen-year-old with type O blood who has been killed in a motorcycle accident. Do they want his liver?

UNOS rules specify that the team has one hour to decide whether or not to accept the organ. This decision is based largely on whether the patient is ready for the liver or if she is in the hospital with an infection or other condition that would preclude transplantation.

The Liver Is Retrieved

If the patient is medically stable and the transplant team agrees to accept the liver, a time will be established to retrieve it. Then a group of liver surgeons rushes off to take out the donor's liver, kidneys, and sometimes the pancreas. Another team usually is sent to collect the same donor's heart and lungs.

After they remove the liver, the surgeons may do a biopsy to ensure that there is no cirrhosis or other damage to the organ. Then they flush the blood from it and place it in preservative solution. After wrapping the liver in sterile plastic and placing it on ice in a cooler, they transport it back to the transplant center. It can be kept outside of a body and remain viable for use for twelve to fifteen hours.

When the Call Comes

As soon as your transplant team decides to accept a donor liver for you, you will be notified. If you are severely ill with fulminant liver disease or liver disease that has deteriorated severely (UNOS status 1 or 2A), you likely will be in a hospital intensive care unit. If you have another UNOS status, you may be in the hospital or at home with a beeper (a pager) when a liver becomes available. If you are not in the hospital and the beeper goes off, you must call the transplant center right away. Your transplant team will give you instructions about when you should be admitted to the hospital (usually four to eight hours later). You shouldn't eat or drink anything from this point on.

PRE-OP

When you get to the hospital, a nurse will take your temperature, pulse, and blood pressure and will check your respiration and weight. You also will undergo a physical exam. Next, an intravenous line will be placed in your arm, and blood will be taken and sent to the laboratory.

If you haven't had a chest X-ray and EKG in the last five days, these tests will be done now.

Just before you are sent to the operating room, your arms, abdomen, and groin will be scrubbed with an antibacterial solution, and you may be given a sedative to help you relax. When you arrive in the operating room, more intravenous and arterial lines will be placed in your arms and neck, and EKG leads will be attached to your chest.

After you have been given anesthesia and you are asleep, an endotracheal tube will be inserted down your throat. This tube is attached to a machine that will help you to breathe during your operation. A soft rubber or plastic tube that goes from your nose to your stomach (a nasogastric tube) or from your mouth to your stomach (an orogastric tube) also will be inserted at this time. This tube will keep your stomach empty and prevent you from vomiting during the operation. Finally, a device called a Foley catheter will be inserted into your urinary bladder to drain urine.

THE OPERATION

Liver transplants are complicated procedures because four blood vessels, plus bile ducts that go from the liver to the intestine, must be severed and reconnected. Liver surgeons use radiographic imaging scans both before and during the operation to accomplish these delicate tasks.

If you have a liver transplant, this is what will happen. The surgeons first will make an incision that is approximately one foot long from one side of your rib cage to the other. Rather than a straight line, this incision is like a three-spoked peace symbol lying on its side. Both your liver and gallbladder will be taken out, and your new liver will be placed in the same anatomical location.

During the operation, several "closed suction" drains will be placed around your new liver to drain excess fluid away from it; this fluid will flow out of tiny holes in your abdomen below the incision. Also, a small cylindrical device called a stent will be placed into the bile duct that carries bile away from the liver. This stent will make it possible for your doctors to monitor the function of your new liver. (It will be removed approximately six weeks after the transplant.)

The whole operation will last approximately 5 and one-half hours (the range is from 4 to 12 hours). Afterward, a member of the surgical team will speak with a member of your family to tell him how the procedure went and when your loved ones will be able to see you.

RECOVERY AND FOLLOW-UP

THE IMMEDIATE POSTOPERATIVE PERIOD

"Almost all patients later say that they felt better the minute they woke up" from surgery, Dr. Pomfret says. After your operation, you will wake up in the intensive care unit (ICU). The breathing (endotracheal) tube probably will be left in place overnight until you can breathe well on your own. Although this tube is not painful, you won't be able to talk until it's removed.

The first day after surgery, you may be moved from the ICU to an inpatient floor of the hospital. Your nasogastric tube probably will come out, and you'll most likely be encouraged to walk around to increase your circulation. During this time, very dedicated nurses and doctors will help you to breathe and get your bowels and fluid levels back to normal. They also will work to regulate your blood pressure (either with drugs called vasopressors for low blood pressure or antihypertensives for high blood pressure). To prevent the development of a lung infection, you will be encouraged to cough regularly and do deep breathing exercises.

About three days after the operation, the urinary catheter and closed suction drains will be removed. When you get the okay to begin eating again, you will be given clear liquids initially and then gradually a low-salt, low-potassium diet. You will be encouraged to eat to build up your strength and help your body to heal. Shortly thereafter, your family members may be allowed to bring your favorite foods to the hospital.

Most transplant patients stay in the hospital for a week or two to regulate the levels of the antirejection medications, or immunosuppressants, that must be taken after this operation.

PROBLEMS THAT MAY OCCUR AFTER YOUR TRANSPLANT

After this major operation, you still may experience some health problems related to your liver. In fact, 10 percent of transplant patients have to go back to the operating room for repair of a bile duct problem, bleeding or blood clot, or infection.

PRIMARY GRAFT NONFUNCTION. Less than 5 to 10 percent of the time, there is primary graft nonfunction, which means that the donor liver simply does not work.

If a new liver fails, it usually does so within a few days of transplantation, and liver specialists can tell that this is occurring because of bleeding, encephalopathy, or very elevated liver function (blood) tests. Unfortunately, the only solution is another transplant operation to replace the nonfunctioning liver with yet another one.

REJECTION EPISODES. Primary graft nonfunction, in which the new liver fails, is not quite the same thing as what doctors call "rejection." Rejection, which occurs in 20 to 40 percent of transplant patients, can include a mild episode of resistance to the new organ or a severe reaction that requires retransplantation.

You may experience what is known as an acute rejection episode. (This can occur at any time, but usually happens within the first six months and most often happens five days to two weeks after the transplant.) If your immune system mounts an attack against this "foreign invader," you may have no symptoms at all, or you may not feel well, you may lose your appetite, and you may have a low-grade fever, abdominal tenderness or increased abdominal fluid, and joint or back pain. You also may feel depressed. Other signs of acute rejection include light-colored stools, dark, cola-colored urine, and jaundice (your skin and the whites of your eyes may look yellow). You may have elevated liver function (blood) tests and a lower output of bile that is light yellow, rather than dark green in color. Your transplant hepatologist will likely want to do a liver biopsy.

Although a rejection episode can be traumatic, more than 95 percent of the time, changing your immunosuppressant medication or adjusting its dosage will resolve this problem, even if you need to be readmitted to the hospital to do so.

BLOOD VESSEL COMPLICATIONS. During a liver transplant, liver surgeons may sever and reconnect up to four major blood vessels. Once in a while, blood clots (thrombosis) may develop in the hepatic artery or portal vein. Your doctor will be able to tell that this is happening because of results of certain laboratory blood tests, radiologic imaging tests, and possibly surgery.

BILE DUCT COMPLICATIONS. If problems occur with the connection of the bile duct to the new liver, your physician may do an X-ray test called a cholangiogram to view the area. This painless technique involves injecting a dye into the stent that was placed during your transplant operation. This will help your doctor to see any leakages or blockages. Usually bile duct problems can be repaired without another operation, although retransplantation sometimes is necessary.

KIDNEY PROBLEMS. Your blood will be tested carefully after the transplant procedure to follow your kidney function. Sometimes because of this long operation, low fluid levels, infection, low blood pressure, or antibiotics and immunosuppressant drugs, the kidneys may lose some functioning ability temporarily. This problem is usually reversible, and treatment depends on the cause of the problem.

INFECTION. After your transplant, you will receive antibiotics to prevent infections. Meticulous hygiene also is very important, and it's a good idea to avoid crowded places and people who have colds and other viral illnesses while you are going through your recuperative period (usually for about three months). If you feel that you are getting a sore throat, cold, or the flu, you should let your doctor know. Also, if you're exposed to a person who has the chicken pox, mumps, or measles, and you've never been infected with the disease, you'll need to contact your physician.

Other than the flu and pneumovax vaccine, which are not live viruses, you should not receive vaccines without your doctor's consent.

If someone in your household is going to be vaccinated with the oral polio vaccine, talk with your doctor.

If you are a woman who uses tampons, you can minimize your risk of infection by changing them often and not using them overnight.

Finally, don't smoke. Doing so can make you even more susceptible to respiratory tract infections.

DISEASE RECURRENCE. Sometimes, unfortunately, certain liver diseases do recur even after a person has had a liver transplant. If you have had a liver transplant because of HBV infection, your risk of disease recurrence is lowest if:

- You had acute, fulminant HBV infection, which destroys many liver cells, so that there is less viral replication.
- You are also infected with the hepatitis D virus (delta virus), which inhibits HBV replication.
- HBV-DNA is low or absent from your blood.
- You take hepatitis B immune globulin (HBIG) before the transplant and for life following the transplant. In fact, most transplant centers now give patients with HBV high doses of intravenous HBIG after this procedure, because studies have shown that this therapy may reduce the HBV recurrence rate by 10 to 40 percent. Unfortunately, the supply of HBIG is limited, and it is expensive (from $15,000 to $60,000 per year).

Immunosuppressant drugs (such as prednisone; cyclosporine; mycophenolate mofetil [Cellcept]; and tacrolimus, or FK-506) given after a liver transplant may enhance viral replication, so many transplant centers stop steroid therapy six to twelve months after transplant. However, preliminary results of some studies show that the drugs lamivudine and famciclovir may prevent HBV recurrence after transplant, because they can inhibit HBV replication.

The recurrence rate of the hepatitis C virus is almost universal after transplantation, in that 90 to 95 percent of the time HCV is present in the patient's bloodstream; 5 percent are lucky and will lose the virus. Although these figures may sound discouraging at first, five years after a liver transplant, most patients who have recurrent HCV will not have severe liver disease or cirrhosis in the new liver.

There is no effective immunoglobulin protection for patients with HCV, as there is for HBV. However, there is reason to be optimistic, because treatment with a combination of the drugs interferon and riba-virin may be helpful for patients who experience recurrent HCV after a liver transplant.

IMMUNOSUPPRESSION

After your liver transplant, you will need to take antirejection drugs, or immunosuppressants, for the rest of your life. Each of the drugs that I'll describe below knock out a certain part of the immune system to prevent it from attacking the new liver. Each drug must be taken at the same time or times every day, and it's very important not to miss a dose. If you do, you should contact your transplant center for guidance.

TACROLIMUS (PROGRAF; ALSO CALLED FK-506). Tacrolimus is a relatively new drug that was cultivated in 1984 from a fungus that grows on a mountainside in Japan. Tacrolimus suppresses the immune system by inhibiting activation of white blood cells called T lymphocytes.

To monitor the amount of this drug in your blood, your blood will be drawn twelve hours after you take it. Your doctor or nurse may refer to the resulting number as a "trough level." The dosage of tacrolimus will be adjusted according to whether this level is too high or too low. In the hospital, you may be given tacrolimus intravenously, but when you go home you will be given tablets.

The side effects of tacrolimus include diabetes and toxicity to the brain (this toxicity causes headaches, temors, and confusion) and kidneys. You also may experience mild to moderate high blood pressure, abdominal cramping, nausea, vomiting, loss of appetite, diarrhea, seizures, tremors, flushing, rash, night sweats, and fatigue.

CYCLOSPORINE (SANDIMMUNE OR, IN A NEWER FORM, NEORAL). Similar to but less potent than tacrolimus, the immunosuppressant cyclosporine, which was discovered in 1972, prevents "T-helper cells" from attacking your new liver by preventing them from developing normally.

In the hospital, you may take cyclosporine in a pill, liquid, or intravenous form. At home, you may take it as a gel cap. You will be told to swallow these capsules, but not to bite or chew them. Just as with tacrolimus, the concentrations of cyclosporine in your blood will be measured frequently. Your dosage will be increased or decreased to prevent drug toxicity (such as temporary kidney or liver damage) from concentrations that are too high or liver rejection from concentrations that are too low.

Side effects of cyclosporine include increased amounts of facial and body hair (hirsutism). Sometimes decreasing the dose of this drug will make this problem go away. Cosmetics, products to get rid of facial hair, or electrolysis also may be used. If you develop this side effect, talk with your doctor. Some patients also experience tremors (which also may disappear with a lower dose); numbness and tingling in the hands, feet, or both; and gum problems.

In addition to these side effects, taking cyclosporine increases your risk of developing high blood pressure (hypertension). If this condition does not improve with a lower dosage of cyclosporine, your physician may prescribe an antihypertensive medication.

Finally, there is a small risk of developing cancer due to immunosuppressive therapy. These cancers include skin (squamous-cell) cancers and cervical cancer, as well as posttransplant lymphoproliferative disorders (PTLD), or lymphoma that develops after a transplant. Taking measures to protect yourself from direct sunlight and, if you are a woman, being diligent about annual screening for cervical cancer are thus very important. Wear sunscreen and be sure to cover your skin with clothing if you are outside for two hours or more. Try to stay out of the sun between 11 A.M. and 2 P.M.

CORTICOSTEROIDS (PREDNISONE, SOLU-MEDROL). Corticosteroids such as prednisone prevent inflammation in the body and alter T cells so that they cannot reject your new liver. In the hospital, you may be given an intravenous form of this drug called Solu-Medrol. When you go home, you will take this drug as a pill with meals, milk, or antacids (never on an empty stomach). Eventually the dosage of prednisone is tapered down to a "maintenance dose," and then you may be able to stop taking it completely.

Many different side effects of prednisone treatment can occur, but these usually decrease as the dosage is reduced. The side effects that you may experience include:

- Facial puffiness (this can be minimized with makeup). Karen Scolaro says, "I will eventually not be on prednisone at all, which my face and I will appreciate greatly."
- Swelling and weight gain because of increased salt and water retention.
- Increased appetite, so a nutritious diet is important. A dietitian may be able to come up with a plan to help you prevent weight gain.
- Acne. Good hygiene and using a medicated soap may be helpful. If this problem becomes bothersome, your doctor may refer you to a dermatologist.
- Facial or body hairiness. Again, you may use cosmetics that bleach or remove facial hair, or you might cover it with a foundation makeup.
- High blood pressure (hypertension).
- Risk of blood sugar problems such as diabetes. Watch for excessive thirst, frequent urination, fatigue, and blurred vision. These problems may decrease when your prednisone dosage is lowered. You may need to take insulin, and if you are a diabetic, your dosage of insulin may need to be increased.
- Bruising.
- Night sweats.
- Muscle weakness in the upper arms and legs. Exercises can help.
- Stomach upset. Taking prednisone with food, milk, or an antacid (to prevent the development of gastric ulcers) is very important. Your doctor also may prescribe a drug such as Pepcid or Maalox to decrease gastric acid secretion and prevent stomach irritation.
- Moodiness. While you are taking prednisone, you may experience mood swings from great happiness to despair. You also may find it difficult to sleep, and you may feel more anxious than usual. Family support is very important at this time.
- Increased risk of infections.
- Eye problems (such as cataracts and glaucoma).

- Increased risk of bone disease (see page 113). Your doctor may recommend that you have bone density measurements done and that you take extra calcium and vitamin D to prevent bone loss from osteoporosis.
- Impaired wound healing. It may take longer to recover from cuts and bruises while you are taking prednisone. Be sure to wash any abrasions well with warm water and soap, then keep cuts dry.

AZATHIOPRINE (IMURAN) OR MYCOPHENOLATE MOFETIL (CELLCEPT). Imuran and Cellcept work by reducing the number of white blood cells called T cells that are available to fight off your new liver. Dr. Elizabeth Pomfret notes that taking such drugs involves "a balancing act" of taking enough immunosuppressants to stay well and yet not so much that one becomes more susceptible to infection. Your doctors will adjust your dosages of these drugs to try to keep your white blood cell counts between 5,000 and 10,000.

The good news about Imuran is that it has less side effects than the other drugs that I've mentioned so far. Just as with prednisone, though, stomach upset can occur, so you may find that taking it after meals helps. You may experience some hair loss (but not balding), too, so you should avoid hair dyes or permanents at this time. Finally, you may develop mouth sores; if you do, your doctor probably will prescribe an antibiotic mouthwash such as mycostatin (Nystatin) or clotrimazole to prevent infection.

Unlike prednisone and Imuran, Cellcept must be taken on an empty stomach. It comes in capsule form, and these capsules should never be crushed or opened.

Side effects of Cellcept include gastrointestinal upset and bleeding, leg pain, weakness, skin rash, and risk of infection. This drug should never be taken while you are also taking cholestyramine or antacids that contain aluminum and magnesium. Doctors also recommend that women use birth control before, during, and six weeks after taking this drug, because animal studies have shown that Cellcept can cause fetal malformations (well-controlled studies have not yet been done in humans).

MEDICINES TO WARD OFF INFECTION

In addition to the all-important immunosuppressants, your transplant team undoubtedly will give you drugs to prevent infection. These may include:

ACYCLOVIR (ZOVIRAX). Acyclovir is given intravenously, by mouth, or as an ointment to manage viral herpes simplex or varicella zoster (shingles). Herpes simplex begins with tingling, pain, itching, and contagious blisters around the mouth or genitals. This virus is present in 8 out of 10 people; it can spring to life when you are under stress or when your immune system is suppressed. The varicella virus can cause shingles. As with herpes simplex, after your initial infection with this virus, the varicella virus waits in the nervous system and becomes active when your immune system is compromised. Acyclovir cannot "cure" either of these viruses, but it can help to manage their symptoms.

The side effects of this drug, when taken intravenously, include headache, tremors, agitation, confusion, and low blood pressure. When it is taken by mouth, its side effects include nausea, diarrhea, and vomiting.

GANCYCLOVIR (CYTOVENE). Gancyclovir is given to manage cytomegalovirus (CMV), which, like herpes simplex and varicella zoster, is a common virus that can come to life when you are taking immunosuppressants. Roughly half of all people in the United States have been infected with this virus, so after your transplant you may be given this antibiotic to lessen your risk of developing CMV disease, which causes flu-like symptoms: fatigue, fever, chills, and body aches.

MYCOSTATIN (NYSTATIN). Another unpleasant infection that can appear while you are taking immunosuppressants is not caused by a virus, but by a fungus, *Candida*. This fungus causes an infection in the mouth that is called thrush.

Nystatin is a yellow mouthwash that can treat this infection. To take this medication, brush your teeth, then swish this mouthwash around in your mouth for a couple of minutes, then swallow it. Most transplant patients use Nystatin for three to six months after their operation.

CLOTRIMAZOLE (MYCELEX). Instead of Nystatin, your physician may prescribe a tablet called clotrimazole to prevent or treat thrush. Instead of a mouthwash, this drug comes in the form of lozenges that you use four to five times every day. Nausea and vomiting are potential side effects of this medicine.

CO-TRIMOXAZOLE, SULFAMETHOXAZOLE-TRIMETHOPRIM (BACTRIM). Finally, in addition to the other medicines that I have mentioned, you may be given Bactrim (liquid or tablets) to prevent pneumonia and other infections after your transplant.

GOING HOME

REGULATING YOUR MEDICATION. After you have been discharged, you may need to stay near the transplant center for a month or more so that the transplant team can monitor your LFTs and your condition as you begin to take immunosuppressants.

TAKING PRECAUTIONS. When you get home, you should contact the transplant center if:

1. You develop a fever of 100.5°F or higher.
2. You have stomach pain, indigestion, nausea, vomiting, or diarrhea.
3. Your urine looks dark yellow or the color of dark tea or cola, or your stools look very light.
4. Your eyes or skin look yellow.
5. You develop pain or increased redness or drainage near your incision or biopsy site.
6. You have symptoms of a cold or the flu.
7. You lose or gain three pounds in one day.
8. You forgot to take your immunosuppressant medication or couldn't take it because you weren't feeling well.
9. You have itching all over your body.

KEEPING FOLLOW-UP APPOINTMENTS. Regular visits to the hospital or clinic for checkups are very important following a liver transplant. You may need to return to the hospital for a visit and lab tests a few days after you go home, then weekly for six to eight weeks, then monthly, and by six months, you may be on an every-two-month schedule. Eventually you may only need to have these appointments twice a year.

During these follow-up visits, blood will be drawn to monitor your liver function. Sometimes an ultrasound or liver biopsy also may be called for.

After your transplant, you may also need to see your dentist every six months and your eye doctor every year. Generally you should not have major dental work done until three months after your liver transplant. If you do have dental work, you most likely will need to take antibiotics ahead of time, and you should check with your doctor and dentist regarding drug interactions with the immunosuppressants (and possibly antibiotics) that you already are taking.

RESUMING EVERYDAY ACTIVITIES. You may need to rest at home for six months or so before returning to work or school. During this time, you may do some light exercises to increase your strength and muscle tone. We recommend walking and climbing stairs for brief (five- to ten-minute) periods. However, don't engage in very physically demanding exercises (such as jogging, bike riding, tennis, or swimming) and avoid heavy lifting for at least two months after your operation.

It's usually safe to resume sexual activity after a liver transplant, although if you are a woman, I would advise you to use contraception for two years after your transplant or until your liver function tests are stable. Talk with your physician about the type of contraception that is most appropriate for you.

Also, talk with your transplant center about when you might drive again. Many of the drugs that you may be taking can have side effects that may affect your ability to operate an automobile safely.

Remember to rest and not push yourself too hard. After all, you've just had major surgery!

> *Every afternoon on my way home from work I stop and have a slush at an ice cream store. The two ladies there know me, and they couldn't believe it was me after the transplant. I wasn't yellow anymore and I didn't look sick. I'd gained more than thirty-five pounds.*
>
> —SCOTT JACKLE

EMERGING THERAPIES

As I have mentioned, the need for donor livers is growing, but the supply of livers has not increased. Because of this great need for livers, more and more living-donor liver transplantation procedures are being done. Scientists also are working diligently to develop other solutions for patients with end-stage liver disease. Let's talk about these promising new therapies.

LIVING DONATION

> I was on the [UNOS] list for two and one-half years, and I started getting very, very sick. And they said I probably was not going to make it in time for a liver to become available.
>
> Dr. Pomfret walked into the room, and she looked at my chart. She introduced herself and she said, "This lady looks like she needs a liver." And that's when she mentioned the living-donor transplant program.
>
> When the idea came up, my first concern was that they might take me off the UNOS list if we agreed to do the operation. And they said no—you'll still be on the list.
>
> Philip decided he was going to save my life. He knew that if they could get me on the table, whether his liver worked or not, I'd have to get a liver.
>
> —KAREN SCOLARO

> If you do the living-donor program and it doesn't work, you get the next liver from the liver bank. So I said to myself, it's a win-win for Karen.
>
> If my liver comes out and doesn't work, it's still going to regenerate. So I'm going to be fine again anyway, but I'm giving her two chances to live. If she rejected both of them, then I'd know that I'd done absolutely everything in my power to help.
>
> —PHILIP SCOLARO

Unfortunately, we don't have "dialysis" for end-stage liver disease like we do for end-stage chronic kidney disease. Patients can wait longer for a kidney transplant, because during this period they can undergo dialysis a few times each week to purge their bodies of toxins that have accumulated.

For patients who otherwise would wait for months or years on the UNOS list (not for patients with acute, fulminant liver failure), one solution is to receive a lobe of liver from a living donor instead. Both portions of the healthy liver then will regenerate within a month or so in both the donor and the recipient.

The donor simply must be in good health and should have a liver that is of an appropriate size to minimize complications (as much as 60 percent of the donor's liver—generally the entire right lobe of this organ—has to be removed to have enough liver tissue to transplant into the recipient). The donor and recipient also should have compatible blood types.

One benefit of such procedures is that patients and surgeons have more control over the timing of the operation, so that instead of rushing to the hospital to receive a liver on short notice, liver recipients can go into the operating room when they are prepared psychologically (and the procedure can be timed so the patient is as physically strong as possible). Being able to schedule this operation also takes some psychological stress off the patient and her family, because generally there is a much shorter wait for the procedure than there is with traditional organ donation.

Finally, another plus of living donation is the knowledge that one person does not have to die in order for another to live.

ADULT-TO-CHILD LIVER TRANSPLANTS. Adult-to-child transplants have been done since 1988. The first known procedure, in which a mother donated part of her liver to her four-year-old daughter, was performed by Dr. Raio and colleagues in Saõ Paulo, Brazil. A year later, in 1989, the first *successful* living donor transplant was performed by Dr. Cristoph Broelsch and colleagues at the University of Chicago. Again, the recipient was a young girl, and her mother was the donor.

Of the estimated 1,000 adult-to-child liver transplants that have been done worldwide, 2 donors have died. One woman experienced a blood clot in her lung (a pulmonary embolism) three days after the transplant operation. Another donor died from a severe and unusual systemic reaction known as an anaphylactic reaction. (To date, there have been very few adult-to-adult donor deaths reported, and the risk of major complications or death for potential liver donors is approximately 1 percent.)

Complications that donors have experienced from these procedures have involved injury to the bile ducts or bile leaks.

ADULT-TO-ADULT LIVER TRANSPLANTS. More and more adult-to-adult liver transplants are now being performed. In the United States, more than 300 such operations have been performed (in Virginia, Miami, Denver, Saint Louis, New York, and Boston). Karen and Philip Scolaro were two of the first people in this country to undergo this procedure. Many more adult-to-adult liver transplants have been performed in Asia, where few people believe in "brain death" and so few people donate their organs. Although organ donation is no longer against the law in Japan, change in these deeply held cultural beliefs has occurred very slowly.

According to Dr. Pomfret, such procedures "will not replace cadaveric transplants by any means." Rather, these procedures hold great potential as a way to deal with the high percentage of patients who die while waiting for a donor liver. She estimates that from one-quarter to one-third of all liver transplants eventually will be done in this manner. In contrast, 40–45 percent of kidney transplants worldwide now involve living donors.

THE OPERATION. The first stage of a living-donor transplant may last as long as five to six hours because surgeons must divide the donor's liver while leaving the blood supply intact. In an adjacent operating room, surgeons then remove the diseased liver of the recipient.

> *We each had our own medical team. He was in one room, and there's a room in the middle where all of the doctors were waiting, and I was in the next room. As soon as they were done with Philip, which actually took a little bit longer than expected, they ran across like little Pacmen.*
>
> —KAREN SCOLARO

After the donor liver is removed, it is generally outside a human body for a much shorter time than the time it takes to transport a liver from a cadaver to the waiting recipient.

The second stage of this procedure, during which the donor liver is placed and sewn into the recipient, may last from four to eight hours, depending on how difficult it is to remove the patient's old liver. Most often the "new" liver will begin working right away, and it will begin to produce bile. Almost half of patients who have just received a new liver can talk to their doctor in the operating room right afterward.

The recovery for patients who have received a new liver by this method is the same as that for patients who have received cadaveric livers.

LIVER-ASSIST DEVICES

We don't have dialysis for patients with severe liver disease, but an artificial liver-assist device is being developed for patients who have fulminant liver failure.

HEPATOCYTE TRANSPLANT

Another promising development for patients who require liver transplants is called a hepatocyte transplant. Fetal liver cells (hepatocytes) are injected into the peritoneal cavity or spleen. When they find their way to the liver, they begin to perform a number of functions such as the production of albumin. This has been achieved in animals, and is currently being studied in human clinical trials.

SUMMARY

It's truly gratifying to witness some of our patients who literally go from the brink of death to lives that are normal and full of vitality after a liver transplant. They soon return to school and work. One has even run the Boston Marathon!

I look forward to further developments in this field. There may be refinements in surgical techniques and better immunosuppression regimens. Furthermore, it is my hope and expectation that soon better therapies will be available to treat the diseases that can lead to advanced liver disease and the need for liver transplantation. In time, as better drugs become available to treat HBV and HCV infections, for example, fewer people will require liver transplants and disease recurrence in those who do will diminish.

Conclusion

If you or someone you care about has liver disease, I hope that you have found this book helpful. I've endeavored to provide you with information about many important aspects of common liver conditions as well as an understanding of how to interpret the results of various tests—such as blood tests, various radiographic investigations, and a liver biopsy—that you may undergo. This knowledge should serve as a solid foundation and empower you to ask the appropriate questions of your physician, do the right things to take care of yourself, and allay many of your concerns and fears.

You should also be encouraged about the progress that has been made so far and about the promising new treatments on the horizon for all types of liver disease. The subspecialty of hepatology evolved only fifty years ago, and several stunning advances have been made since then. Major breakthroughs include the identification of the various forms of viral hepatitis; the development of sensitive and reliable blood assays for identifying and quantitating the hepatitis B and C virus; the introduction of very effective vaccines for the prevention of hepatitis A and B viral infection; the invention of an array of innovative radiologic imaging studies; advances in liver surgery; performance of liver transplantation; and the exciting evolution of treatments for many chronic liver disorders.

Although many liver disorders still occur in epidemic proportions worldwide, it is indeed a most gratifying and rewarding time to be a hepatologist, for we can now diagnose and effectively treat many liver conditions, and rapid strides in the art and science of medicine are made literally every week. As a specialist who has had the privilege to have worked for a quarter of a century taking care of patients, teaching, writing, lecturing, and doing clinical research, I learn every single day from my patients, students, and colleagues.

Almost certainly, your liver specialist is also learning about the new therapies available to treat many common liver disorders. The first meeting of the American Association for the Study of Liver Diseases was held in Chicago in 1950. From a handful of visionary and dedicated physicians, this association has grown enormously, so that now as many as three to four thousand physicians from all over the world attend this annual meeting to discuss the latest developments in the field. I always come away from this meeting armed with the knowledge that young and brilliant (and also old and wise!) clinicians and investigators are developing effective, safe, and inexpensive vaccines; animal models of human liver disease; and gene therapy and other novel treatments. Recently there have also been noteworthy improvements in the field of liver transplantation.

Thus, whether you are about to embark on a course of treatment for your liver disease or you have been treated for a liver condition for some time, let me assure you that there is every reason to look forward to the future with great hope and bright optimism.

Notes to Selected Articles Described in the Text

· ·

Bean, W. B. *Vascular Spiders and Related Lesions of the Skin*. Oxford, England: Blackwell Scientific Publications, 1959.

Belle, S. H., K. C. Beringer, and K. M. Detre. "Liver Transplantation for Alcoholic Liver Disease in the United States: 1988 to 1995." *Liver Transplantation and Surgery* 3, no. 3 (1997): 212–19.

Ewing, C. "Detecting Alcoholism: The CAGE Questionnaire." *JAMA* 252 (1984): 1905–07.

Gerts, A., and V. Rogiers. "Sho-saiko-to: The Right Blend of Traditional Oriental Medicine and Liver Cell Biology." *Hepatology* 29 (1999): 282.

Marcellin, P., N. Boyer, A. Gervais, et al. "Long-term Histologic Improvement and Loss of Detectable Intrahepatic HCV RNA in Patients with Chronic Hepatitis C and Sustained Response to Interferon-alpha Therapy." *Annals of Internal Medicine* 127 (1997): 875–81.

National Institute on Alcohol Abuse and Alcoholism. *Alcohol Alert No. 19: Alcohol and the Liver*. Pamphlet 329. Rockville, Md.: National Institute on Alcohol Abuse and Alcoholism, 1993.

Poynard, T., P. Bedossa, and P. Opolon. "Natural History of Liver Fibrosis Progression in Patients with Chronic Hepatitis C." *Lancet* 349 (1997): 825–32.

Zimmerman, Hyman J. *Drug-induced Liver Injury Clinical*. Syllabus for postgraduate course, "Clinical and Pathological Correlations in Liver Disease: Approaching the Next Millennium." American Association for the Study of Liver Diseases, 1998.

Resources

· ·

NATIONAL ORGANIZATIONS

The American Liver Foundation
1425 Pompton Ave., Cedar Grove, NJ 07009-1000
Tel.: (201) 256-2550; fax: (201) 256-3214
Hotlines (toll-free): (800) GO-LIVER (465-4837) and (888) 4HEP-ABC
  (443-7222)

Digestive Health Initiative Viral Hepatitis Education Campaign
Tel.: (301) 654-2635

The Hep C Connection
1177 Grant St., Suite 200
Denver, CO 80203
Tel.: (303) 860-0800
Hotline (toll-free): (800) 522-HEPC; help line: (800) 390-1202

The Hepatitis C Foundation
1502 Russett Dr.
Warminster, PA 18974-1176
Tel.: (215) 672-2606; (toll-free): (800) 324-7305; fax: (215) 672-1518
Hotline (toll-free): (800) 324-7305

The Hepatitis Foundation International
30 Sunrise Terrace
Cedar Grove, NJ 07009-1423
Tel.: (973) 239-1035; toll-free: (800) 891-0707; fax: (973) 857-5044

Transplant Recipient International Organization (TRIO)
1735 Eye St. NW, Suite 917
Washington, DC 20006
Tel.: (202) 293-0980

United Network for Organ Sharing (UNOS)
1100 Boulders Parkway
Suite 500
P.O. Box 13770
Richmond, VA 23225-8770
Tel.: (804) 330-8500; toll-free (888) TX-INFO1 (894-6361)

U.S. GOVERNMENT AGENCIES

NATIONAL AGENCIES

Centers for Disease Control and Prevention (CDC)
Hepatitis Branch, Mailstop G37
Division of Viral and Rickettsial Diseases
National Center for Infectious Diseases
Centers for Disease Control and Prevention
1600 Clifton Road, NE
Atlanta, GA 30333
Tel. (toll-free): (800) 311-3435; (888) 4HEPCDC (443-7232)
Hotline: (404) 332-4555

Food and Drug Administration
Office of Consumer Affairs
HFE 88
5600 Fishers Lane
Rockville, MD 20857
Tel.: (800) 532-4440

National Council on Alcoholism and Drug Dependence (NCADD)
12 West 21st St., 7th Floor
New York, NY 10010
Tel.: (212) 206-6770; fax (212) 645-1690; toll-free: (800) NCA-CALL
   [800-622-2255]

The National Institutes for Health (NIH)
Bethesda, MD 20892

> *National Cancer Institute (NCI)*
> Office of Cancer Communications
> Building 31, Room 10A07
> 31 Center Drive MSC 2580
> Bethesda, MD 20892-2580
> Tel.: (301) 496-5583; toll-free: (800) 4-CANCER (422-6237)

National Institute on Alcohol Abuse and Alcoholism (NIAAA)
Suite 409, Willco Building
6000 Executive Blvd.
MSC 7003
Bethesda, MD 20892-7003
Tel.: (301) 443-3860

National Insititute of Allergy and Infectious Diseases (NIAID)
NIAID Office of Communications
Building 31, Room 7A-50
31 Center Dr., MSC 2520
Bethesda, MD 20892-2520
Tel.: (301) 496-5717

National Institute of Diabetes & Digestive & Kidney Diseases (NIDDK)
National Digestive Diseases Information Clearinghouse (ND-DIC)
2 Information Way
Bethesda, MD 20892-3570

U.S. Department of Health and Human Services Division of Transplantation
5600 Fishers Lane, Room 7-29
Rockville, MD 20857
Tel.: (301) 443-7577

LOCAL AGENCIES

To learn more about hepatitis infections in your state, call your state department of public health, epidemiology division.

DRUG TRIALS AND FINANCIAL ASSISTANCE

Amgen (manufactures Infergen)
Reimbursement Services
Tel. (toll-free): (888) 508-8088

Hoffman La Roche (manufactures Roferon-A interferon)
Medical Needs Program
340 Kingsland St.
Nutley, NJ 07110
Tel. (toll-free): (888) 300-PATH or (800) 285-4484

Schering-Plough Corp. (manufactures Intron-A and Rebetron)
Tel. (toll-free) (800) 521-7157 (ext. 147 for financial assistance program)

WEB SITES

Several sites related to liver diseases are available on the Internet. They sometimes contain inaccurate information, however, so always check with your doctor before trying any of the therapies that you read about. I do not specifically endorse any of the Web sites listed below.

The American Liver Foundation
http://www.liverfoundation.org
e-mail: info@liverfoundation.org

American Share Foundation
http://www.asf.org

The Hep C Connection
http://www.hepc-connection.org
e-mail: hepc-connection@worldnet.att.net

The Hepatitis C Foundation
http://www.hepcfoundation.org

Hepatitis Foundation
http://www.hepfi.org

Hepatitis Information Network
http://www.hepnet.com

Heponline.net
http://www.heponline.net

Iron Overload Disease Association Inc. (Hemochromatosis)
http://www.ironoverload.org

NCADD
http://www.ncadd.org

NIAID
http://www.niaid.nih.gov

NIDDK
http://www.niddk.nih.gov
e-mail: nddic@aerie.com

Organ Transplant Fund, Inc.
http://www.otf.org

Index

· ·

abdominal pain, 67, 108, 127, 213, 222
abdominal swelling. *See* ascites.
acetaldehyde, 7, 117, 119–20
acetaminophen, 123–24, 125
acupuncture, 61, 97
acyclovir, 42, 261
AdoMet, 145
alanine transaminase (ALT), 12, 27, 47,
    59, 74–75, 88, 89, 90, 91, 93,
    105, 106, 109, 182, 201
albumin, 4, 13, 76, 109, 154, 182, 243,
    248
alcohol ablation, 230–31
alcohol consumption, 7, 34, 57, 117,
    118, 123, 208
alcoholic hepatitis, 21, 120, 131–44, 157
alcoholic liver disease, xi, 34, 77, 117–46
    alcoholic hepatitis, 21, 120, 131–44,
        157
    fatty liver disease, 126–31
    and hepatoma, 144
    and iron overload, 209
    liver transplants for, 143–44
    research on, 145–46
    risk factors for, 118–26
    See also cirrhosis.
Alcoholics Anonymous (AA), 137, 139,
    140, 155
alcoholism
    and anemia, 172
    biological basis for, 138–39
    and cirrhosis, 144, 155–56
    drug therapy for, 137–38, 139
    and hepatoma risk, 226

nutritional counseling for, 141–42
recovery programs, 129–31, 136–37,
    139–41
and risk factors, 118, 119, 121–22,
    143
Aldomet, 108
alendronate, 113
alkaline phosphatase, 12–13, 76, 182,
    217
alpha-fetoprotein (AFP) test, 14, 34,
    76–77, 79, 173–74, 217, 222,
    228
alphalanritrypsin deficiency, 158, 226
ALT. *See* alanine transaminase.
Alter, Harvey, 50
alternative treatments, 95–99
amantadine, 93
American Association for the Study of
    Liver Disease, 96, 101
American Liver Foundation, 94
American Red Cross, 59, 60
ammonia, 5, 7, 11, 170
anemia, 12, 14, 35, 131
    and cirrhosis, 172
    hemolytic, 10, 86
    iron deficiency, 80, 191, 195
    and iron overload, 209
angiogenesis, 90, 231
Antabuse, 138
antibodies, HAV, 24
antilymphocyte serum (ALS), 236
antimitochondrial antibody (AMA), 14,
    182
antinuclear antibody (ANA), 14, 107

antioxidants, 97
appetite loss
    alcoholic liver disease, 127, 132
    autoimmune hepatitis, 105, 108
    cirrhosis, 68, 152
    liver tumors, 213
    Rebetron therapy, 87
    viral hepatitis, 27, 31, 47, 49
arthritis, and hemochromatosis, 197
ascites, 18, 31, 45, 47, 69, 78, 109, 114,
        132, 152, 154, 164–67, 179,
        204, 214, 243, 248
aspartate transaminase (AST), 12, 27, 47,
        74–75, 105, 106, 109, 201
aspirin, 124, 169
AST. See aspartate transaminase.
autoimmune disorders, 180, 188
autoimmune hepatitis, 14, 22, 105–16,
        173
    complications of, 111–12, 157
    diagnosis of, 105–07, 109–10
    drug therapy for, 112–15
    incidence of, 108
    and liver transplants, 115
    and lupus, 107, 108, 115
    mild to severe, 110–11
    risk factors for, 107–08
    symptoms of, 108–09
azathioprine, 112, 113–14, 260

bacteria, and liver function, 7
Bactrim, 262
balloon tamponade, 169
Baxter Healthcare Corporation, 59
Bean, William Bennett, 133
Beethoven, Ludwig von, 165
benzodiazepines, 137–38
beta-carotene, 97
bile, 2, 4–5
bile acids, 6
biliary atresia, 160–61
bilirubin, 4, 5–6, 13, 76, 105, 109, 134,
        154, 182, 214, 243, 248
biochemical response, 88

biopsy. See liver biopsy.
birth control pills, and liver tumors,
        221–23, 224
bleeding
    alcoholic hepatitis, 132
    and blood-clotting impairment, 153,
        169
    congestive gastropathy, 182, 191
    liver biopsy, 135, 153
    liver tumors, 221, 222
    See also variceal bleeding.
blood-clotting factors, 4, 13, 75, 153,
        169, 243
bloodletting. See phlebotomy.
blood sugar, and liver function, 6
blood tests, 11–14
    alcoholic liver disease, 127–28,
        133–34
    autoimmune hepatitis, 106–07,
        109–10
    of blood donors, 59–60, 69
    cirrhosis, 152
    cirrhosis (primary biliary), 181–83
    hemochromatosis, 202–04
    hepatitis A, 27, 205
    hepatitis B, 31–32, 205
    hepatitis C, 71–77
    hepatitis D, 47, 49
    liver tumors, 34, 216–17
    for viral inhibition, 41–42
blood transfusion
    and hepatitis transmission, 50, 55,
        58–60, 69
    and iron overload, 195, 209
    and transfusion-transmitted virus
        (TTV), 54
blood urea nitrogen (BUN), 134
body piercing, and hepatitis C
        transmission, 61
bone loss, 113, 158, 180, 189–90
bone marrow suppression, and interferon
        therapy, 35, 38–39
breast enlargement, male, 10, 69, 152
breast-feeding, and hepatitis C, 64

breath odor, 11
Broelsch, Cristoph, 265

calcium deposits, 191
calcium supplements, 113, 189, 190
Caplan, Arthur, 238
carbohydrate metabolism, and liver
    function, 6
cardiac cirrhosis, 161
CAT scan, 15, 27–28, 79, 153, 154, 173,
    204, 218
celiac sprue, 76, 180, 191
Cellcept, 260
Centers for Disease Control (CDC), 25,
    49, 56, 58, 157
chaparral leaf, 99
chemotherapeutic embolization, 229–30
children
    hepatitis A, 24, 25
    hepatitis B, 30
    liver transplants, 242–43, 265–66
Childs-Pugh classification, 154, 168
cholangiogram, 255
cholecystitis, acute, 16–17
cholestatic hepatitis, 27, 28, 76
cholesterol, 6, 180, 183
cholesterol deposits, 190
cholestyramine, 186
cirrhosis, 147–74
    and alcoholism, 129, 155–56
    and autoimmune hepatitis, 109, 114,
        115
    causes of, 155–63
    complications of, 109, 164–74
    deaths from, 144
    diagnosis of, 19, 23, 147–49, 152–
        54, 205
    and family screening, 163–64
    and hepatitis B, 30, 32, 34, 156
    and hepatitis C, 57, 68, 69, 79,
        147–48, 156, 225
    and hepatitis D, 45, 47, 156
    and hepatoma, 226
    incidence of, 118

and iron overload, 157, 195, 198,
    202
and liver cancer (hepatoma), 173–74,
    184
and liver transplant, 241
severity of, 154–55, 230–31
symptoms of, 68–69, 148, 151–52,
    179–80
treatment of, 149–50
cirrhosis, primary biliary (PBC), xi, 5, 12,
    14, 108, 173, 175–93
    diagnosis of, 181–83
    and hepatoma, 184
    and liver transplant, 187, 190, 192,
        241–42
    risk factors for, 176
    stages of, 184
    symptoms of, 177–81
    treatment of, 158–59, 185–92
clotrimazole, 262
cocaine snorting, and hepatitis C
    transmission, 64–65
colchicine, 185
colestipol, 186
comfrey, 99
complete blood count (CBC), 11–12, 75,
    181–82, 216
computed axial tomography. *See* CAT
    scan.
congestive gastropathy, 182, 191
Conn, Harold, 165
corticosteroids, 34, 47
    and alcoholic hepatitis, 142
    and autoimmune hepatitis, 110–11,
        112–14
    and hepatitis B, 34
    and hepatitis D, 47
    and immunosuppression, 258–60
    side effects of, 113, 157, 259–60
creatine phosphokinase (CPK) test, 75
CRST syndrome, 180, 191
cryoglobulinemia syndrome, essential
    mixed, 67–68
cryosurgery, 229

CT scan. *See* CAT scan.
C-282-Y mutation test, 203–04
cyclosporine, 115, 257–58
cytomegalovirus (CMV), 261
Cytovene, 42, 261

delta hepatitis. *See* hepatitis D (delta)
    virus (HDV).
depression
    and alcoholism, 121–22
    and interferon therapy, 39
dermatomyositis, 180, 192
desferoxymine, 208
DEXA (dual-energy X-ray
    absorptiometry), 189
diabetes, 197, 201, 222
diagnosis, 9–20
    alcoholic hepatitis, 133–36
    ascites, 164–65
    autoimmune hepatitis, 105–07,
        109–10
    cirrhosis, 19, 23, 147–49, 152–54,
        205
    cirrhosis (primary biliary), 181–83
    and family screenings, 163–64, 208
    fatty liver disease, 126–29
    hemochromatosis, 194, 198–206
    hepatic encephalopathy, 170–71
    hepatitis A, 27–28, 205
    hepatitis B, 31–33, 205
    hepatitis C, 69–80
    hepatitis D, 47
    hepatitis E, 49
    hepatoma, 214–20, 227–28, 232
    liver cancer (metastatic), 233
    liver tumors (benign), 214–20, 221,
        222, 223–24
    and medical history, 10, 214–16
    signs and symptoms in, 10–11, 133
    variceal bleeding, 19, 20, 80, 136, 168
    See also blood tests; endoscopy;
        imaging tests; liver biopsy;
        physical examination.
diarrhea, 179, 187–88, 191

diet and nutrition
    and alcoholism, 122, 141–42
    and hepatic encephalopathy, 171
    and hepatitis C, 93–94, 97
    and iron overload, 209
disulfiram, 138
diuretics, 166
Dr. Maddrey's Formula, 135, 142
drug abuse
    cocaine snorting, 64–65
    intravenous, 24, 26, 58, 69
    See also alcoholism.
drug therapy
    acetaminophen in, 123–24, 125
    for alcohol addiction, 137–38, 139
    for alcoholic hepatitis, 142–43
    for autoimmune hepatitis, 112–15
    for cirrhosis (primary biliary),
        158–59, 185
    for hepatitis B, 34–43
    for hepatitis C, 45, 81–82, 83–92, 93,
        101–03
    for hepatitis D, 47–48
    for hepatoma, 231
    herbal remedies, 96, 97, 98, 99
    for itching, 186
    after liver transplants, 256–57, 257–62
    for variceal bleeding, 20, 136, 168
    See also side effects of drug therapy;
        specific drugs.
drug toxicity, 7–8, 12
dry gland syndrome, 109, 188

ELISA tests, 71
emotional support, 94
endocrine disorders, and
    hemochromatosis, 197
endoscopic band ligation, 114, 168–69,
    210
endoscopic retrograde cholangiopacreato-
    graphy (ERCP), 16
endoscopic sclerotherapy, 168
endoscopy, 19–20, 80, 114, 136,
    168–69, 205

environmental toxins, and hepatoma, 226–27
enzyme-linked immunosorbent assay (ELISA), 71
erythropoietin, 216
estrogen, 189–90
exercise, 113
eye problems, and interferon therapy, 40

falciform ligament, 4
famciclovir, 42–43
family screenings, 163–64, 208
fatigue
    alcoholic liver disease, 132
    autoimmune hepatitis, 105, 108, 114
    cirrhosis, 68, 152, 198
    cirrhosis (primary biliary), 158, 178
    interferon therapy, 35, 38
    liver tumors, 213
    viral hepatitis, 31, 47, 67
fatty liver disease, 126–31
ferritin, 203
fever, 26, 49, 131
fibrolamellar hepatoma, 232
fibromyalgia, and hepatitis C, 68
FK-506, 115, 257
"flapping tremor," 11
fluid retention. *See* ascites.
flu-like symptoms
    autoimmune hepatitis, 105
    hepatitis C, 57
    interferon therapy, 37–38
fluoride, 113
focal nodular hyperplasia (FNH), 16, 223–25
Folkman, Judah, 90
food contamination, 23–24
Food and Drug Administration (FDA), 30, 84, 124
Fosamax, 113

gallbladder, 2
gallstones, 180, 189

Gammagard, 59
gamma globulin prophylaxis, 25
gancyclovir, 42, 261
gastroenterologist, 20, 32–33, 70, 83, 99, 110, 131–32
gender, and alcoholic liver disease, 120
genetic factors
    in alcoholic liver disease, 119–20, 143
    and family screening, 163–64, 208
    in hemochromatosis, 196, 208
    in hepatitis C, 14, 73
genotype test, for hepatitis C, 14, 73
germander, 99
Global Alliance for Vaccines and Immunizations, 234
glycogen storage disease, 161, 222
gordolobo herbal tea, 99
Gordon, Fredric, 241
Groopman, Jerome, 100–101
guided imagery, 97
gums, bleeding, 132
gynecomastia, 10

HAV antibody test, 14
HBsAg test, 31
HBV core antibody test, 14
HBV surface antigen test, 14
HCV antibody tests, 59, 60, 64, 71, 72
HCV-RNA-PCR test, 14, 72–73, 88, 91
heart problems, and hemochromatosis, 198
hemangioma, 78
hematocrit, 35, 84
hemochromatosis, xi, 77, 126, 135, 144, 157
    diagnosis of, 194, 198–206
    and hepatoma risk, 226
    and liver transplant, 242
    related disorders, 196–98
    risk factors for, 196
    symptoms of, 196
    treatment of, 206–08
hemolytic anemia, 10, 86

hepactectomy, partial, 229
hepatic adenoma, 190, 221–23
hepatic artery, 2
hepatic encephalopathy, 11, 94, 106–07,
    109, 133, 138, 154, 167, 180
    diagnosis of, 170–71
    and liver transplants, 241, 243, 248
    symptoms of, 170
    treatment of, 171
hepatic hemangioma, 220–21
hepatic osteodystrophy, 189, 243
hepatic scintiscanning, 16
hepatitis
    alcoholic, 21, 120, 131–44, 157
    and blood transfusion, 50
    cholestatic, 27, 28, 76
    drug-induced, 21–22, 32
    fulminant, 109
    See also alcoholic liver disease;
        autoimmune hepatitis; viral
        hepatitis.
hepatitis A virus (HAV), 22, 23–29
    antibodies to, 24, 27
    diagnosis of, 14, 27–28, 205
    overview, 51
    risk factors for, 23–24, 106
    spread of, 28–29
    symptoms of, 26–27
    treatment of, 28
    vaccine for, xii, 24–26, 157
hepatitis B immune globulin (HBIG), 30
hepatitis B virus (HBV), xi, 17, 22, 26,
    29–44, 225
    and alcohol consumption, 122,
        128–29
    chronic carriers, 29
    and cirrhosis, 30, 32, 34, 156
    diagnosis of, 14, 31–33, 205
    hepatitis D piggybacking, 32, 41, 44, 45
    overview, 51
    risk factors for, 29–30
    spread of, 33
    symptoms of, 31
    treatment of, 33–44

    vaccine for, xii, 29, 30, 46, 157, 234
hepatitis C virus (HCV)
    acute, 56–57
    and alcohol consumption, 122, 128–
        29, 130–31
    chronic, 22, 56, 57
    and cirrhosis, 57, 68, 69, 79, 147–48,
        156, 225
    deaths from, 56
    diagnosis of, 14, 69–80
    incidence of, xi, 44–45, 55, 56, 235
    and iron overload, 195, 209
    mild, 81–82
    overview, 52
    recurrence after transplant, 256–57
    risk factors for, 57–65
    symptoms of, 66–69
    treatment of
        alternative treatments, 95–99
        diet, 93–94, 97
        drug therapy, 45, 81–82, 83–92,
            93, 101–03
        emotional support in, 94
        future prospects for, 100–101
        phlebotomy, 68, 77, 92–93
    vaccine for, 100
hepatitis D (delta) virus, 22, 45–48
    diagnosis of, 47
    hepatitis B piggyback, 32, 41, 44, 45
    overview, 52
    prevention of, 46
    symptoms of, 46–47
    treatment of, 47–48
hepatitis E virus (HEV), 22, 48–50, 53
hepatitis F virus, 50
hepatitis G virus (HGV), 50
hepatitis viral serological markers, 14
hepatocellular injury, 12
hepatocytes, 4
hepatocyte transplant, 265
hepato-iminodiacetic acid (HIDA) scan,
    16–17
hepatologist, 20, 32–33, 34, 36, 42, 70,
    83, 99, 110, 115

Hepatology, 96
hepatoma (fibrolamellar), 232
hepatoma (primary liver cancer), 14, 50,
    212, 225–31
   and alcoholic liver disease, 144
   and autoimmune hepatitis, 111
   and cirrhosis, 173–74, 184
   diagnosis of, 214–20, 227–28
   and hemochromatosis, 205–06
   and hepatitis B, 30, 225
   and hepatitis C, 76, 225
   incidence of, 225–26
   and liver transplant, 242
   prognosis for, 227
   risk factors for, 226–27
   screening for, 34, 76–77, 78–79, 213
   symptoms of, 214, 227
   treatment of, 228–31
hepatopulmonary syndrome, 172–73
hepatorenal syndrome, 172
herbal medication, 96, 97, 98, 99
HIDA scan, 16–17
histologic response, 88–89
Hogan, John, 121, 130, 131, 140–41
Hoofnagle, Jay, 92
Houghton, Michael, 44
hypertension, portal, 165
hypoalbuminemia, 243
hypothyroidism, 176, 180, 188

ibuprofen, 124
IgM anti-HAV antibody test, 27
IgM core antibody test, 31, 32
imaging tests, 15–17, 77–79, 126,
    153–54, 173, 204, 217–19, 222,
    223, 228
immunoglobulin G (IgG) level, 107
immunosuppressant drugs, xii, 115, 256,
    257–60
Imuran, 112, 113–14, 260
Inderal, 20, 80, 136, 168
induction therapy, 101
infection
   and hemochromatosis, 197

and liver transplant, 255–56, 261–62
inflammatory bowel disease, 76, 159
interferon, 32, 34–42, 47–48
   in Rebetron therapy, 45, 73, 81,
    83–84
   refinements to, 101
   side effects of, 35, 37–40
interleukin-10 (IL-10), 102
intrahepatic cholestasis of pregnancy, 12,
    178
intravenous drug use, 24, 26, 58, 69
iron deficiency anemia, 14, 80, 191,
    195
iron overload, 6–7, 14, 77
   causes of, 195, 208–10
   See also hemochromatosis.
iron reduction therapy. *See* phlebotomy.
isoniazid (INH), 108
itching, 10, 68
   cholestatic liver disease, 27, 28, 76
   cirrhosis, 158, 175, 177–78, 185–87,
    198
   Rebetron therapy, 86
   treatment of, 185–87

Jackle, Scott, 239, 250, 263
jaundice, 10, 11, 16
   alcoholic hepatitis, 131, 132, 134
   autoimmune hepatitis, 105, 106
   cirrhosis, 152, 198, 243
   cirrhosis (primary biliary), 178–79
   hepatitis A, 27
   hepatitis B, 31
   hepatitis C, 57, 68, 76, 78
   hepatitis D, 47
   hepatitis E, 49
   liver cancer (metastatic), 232–33
   liver tumors, 213, 214
jin bu huan, 99
joint pain, 31, 67, 108, 114, 180
Judd, Naomi, 96–97

ketoprofen, 124
kidney failure, 133, 134, 172

kidney function
    and liver transplant, 255
    tests, 134
Kupffer cells, 7

lactate dehydrogenase (LDH), 13, 217
lactulose, 171
lamivudine, 42, 48
laparoscopy/laparotomy, 19
Leshner, Alan, 138
leukemoid reaction, 134
levamisole, 34
LeVeen shunt, 166
libido loss, and Rebetron therapy, 87–88
Lieber, Charles S., 145
liver
    blood supply to, 2
    composition of, 4
    enlarged, 27, 47, 49, 105, 106, 126,
        131
    functions of, 4–8, 169, 170
    location of, 2, 3
    personality traits associated with, 1
    size of, 2
liver biopsy, 80, 110, 126–27, 128, 228
    complications of, 134–35, 153
    and liver tumors, 219–20
    needle, 17–18, 32–33, 78, 153, 183,
        204
    questions to ask doctor, 135–36
    surgical, 19
    transvenous, 18–19
liver cancer
    metastatic, 232–33
    See also hepatoma (primary liver
        cancer).
liver enzyme tests, 12–13, 27, 41, 42,
        74–75, 109
liver failure, fulminant, 242, 243
liver function tests (LFTs), 12–13, 19,
        74–77, 126, 127–28, 152, 203,
        216–17, 222
liver-spleen scan, 16, 219
liver transplants, xii, 28, 235–68

acceptance criteria, 248–49
and alcoholic liver disease, 143–44
and autoimmune hepatitis, 115
candidates for, 240–44
and cirrhosis (primary biliary), 187,
        190, 192
contraindications, 244–45
evaluation process, 245–48
and hepatitis B, 43–44
and hepatitis C, 82–83, 235
and hepatitis D, 48
hepatocyte, 265
and hepatoma, 229
history of, 236–37
living-donor, 235, 247–48, 264–67
operation, 250–53
organ allocation, 237–40
recovery/follow-up, 253–63
waiting period, 249–50
liver tumors (benign), 211–34
    diagnosis of, 214–20, 221, 222, 223–24
    discovery of, 212–13, 222
    focal nodular hyperplasia, 223–25
    hepatic adenoma, 221–23
    hepatic hemangioma, 220–21
    and liver transplant, 242
    symptoms of, 213–14, 221, 222, 223
    treatment of, 221, 222–23, 224–25
liver tumors (malignant)
    fibrolamellar hepatoma, 232
    See also hepatoma (primary liver cancer).
living-donor transplants, 235, 247–48,
        264–67
lobucavir, 42
Love Can Build a Bridge (Judd), 97
lupus erythematosus, systemic (SLE),
        107, 108, 115
lymph nodes, enlarged, 27

magnetic resonance angiography (MRA),
        16, 218
magnetic resonance
    cholangiopacreatography
        (MRCP), 16

magnetic resonance imaging (MRI), 15–16, 79, 204, 218–19
Mallory's hyaline, 159
malnutrition, and alcoholic liver disease, 122
manic-depression, and alcoholism, 121–22
margosa oil, 99
Martin, Maureen, 238, 240
massage, 97
maté tea, 99
medical history, 10, 214–16
medications. *See* drug therapy; side effects of drug therapy.
meditation, 96, 97
mental confusion. *See* hepatic encephalopathy.
methotrexate, 158, 185
methyldopa, 108
Miacalcin, 113
milk thistle, 99, 102
mofetil, 260
MRA (magnetic resonance angiography), 16
MRCP (magnetic resonance cholangiopacreatography), 16
MRI (magnetic resonance imaging), 15–16, 79, 204, 218–19
Murphy, Christine, 105–06
Mycelex, 262
mycostatin, 261

naltrexone, 139
NASH. *See* nonalcoholic steatohepatitis.
National Hospital Discharge Survey, 144
National Institute on Alcohol Abuse and Alcoholism, 118
National Institutes of Health (NIH), 42, 92, 100–101, 237
National Organ Transplant Act (NOTA), 237, 238
nausea
    alcoholic liver disease, 127, 132
    autoimmune hepatitis, 114

cirrhosis, 68, 152, 198
    liver tumors, 213
    Rebetron therapy, 87
    viral hepatitis, 31, 47
needle biopsy, 17–18, 33, 78, 153, 183, 204
needle punctures, accidental, 65, 72
neomycin, 171
nephrotic syndrome, 76
nitrofurantoin, 108
nonalcoholic steatohepatitis (NASH), xi, 17, 22, 77, 159–60, 173
nonsteroidal anti-inflammatory agents (NSAIDS), 124, 169
nosebleeds, 132, 169
numbness and tingling, 67
nutrition. *See* diet and nutrition.
nutritional supplements, 94, 97, 145, 187
Nystatin, 261

obesity
    and alcoholic liver disease, 122
    and nonalcoholic steatohepatitis, 160
oral-anal sexual activity, 24
oral contraceptives, and liver tumors, 221–23, 224
organ transplants. *See* liver transplants; transplants.
osteomalacia, 189
osteoporosis, 180, 189–90
ovulation cycle, disruption of, 69, 152

pain relievers, and alcoholic liver disease risk, 123–26
paracentesis, 164, 166
PCR test. *See* HCV-RNA-PCR test.
pentoxifylline, 145, 146
percutaneous transhepatic cholangiography (PTC), 16
peritonitis, spontaneous bacterial, 132
phlebotomy, 68, 77, 92–93, 160, 206–07
phototherapy, for itching, 186
Phyllanthus amarus, 34

physical examination, 10–11, 27, 70,
    105–06, 127, 131, 133, 152,
    181, 202, 216
pilocarpine (Salagen), 188
plasmapheresis, 187, 190
platelets, 35, 88, 182
polyethylene glycol (PEG) interferon, 101
polymerase chain reaction (PCR) test, 50,
    62
polyunsaturated lecithin (PUL), 145
Pomfret, Elizabeth, 247, 250, 253, 260,
    266
porphyria cutanea tarda, 68, 77, 195,
    210
portocaval shunt, 195, 210
post-traumatic stress syndrome, and
    alcoholism, 121
prednisone, 28, 110–11, 112–13, 114,
    142, 258
  side effects of, 113, 259–60
pregnancy
  hepatitis B screening during, 30
  hepatitis transmission to newborn, 30,
    63–64
  intrahepatic cholestasis of, 12, 178
  Rebetron side effects in, 84
primary biliary cirrhosis (PBC). See
    cirrhosis, primary biliary.
primary graft nonfunction, 254
primary hepatocellular carcinoma. See
    hepatoma (primary liver cancer).
primary liver cancer. See hepatoma
    (primary liver cancer).
primary sclerosing cholangitis (PSC), 12,
    159, 241
propranolol, 20, 80, 136, 168
protease inhibitors, 102
protein in diet, 94, 171
protein-losing enteropathy, 76
prothrombin time (PT), 13, 75, 105, 106,
    134, 135, 153, 182, 244, 248
pruritis. See itching.
PTC (percutaneous transhepatic
    cholangiography), 16

radiofrequency ablation (RFA), 231
radiologic tests. See imaging tests.
Raio, Dr., 265
Raynaud's disease, 191
Rebetron therapy, 45, 73, 81,
    83–92
  side effects of, 85–88
recombinant immunoblast assay (RIBA),
    71, 72
rectal bleeding, 47, 167
red blood count, 12, 35, 222
rejection episodes, 254–55
rheumatologist, 192
RIBA test, 71, 72
ribavirin, 45, 73, 81
  See also Rebetron therapy.
risk factors
  alcoholic liver disease, 118–26
  autoimmune hepatitis, 107–08
  cirrhosis, 155–63
  cirrhosis (primary biliary), 176
  hemochromatosis, 196
  hepatitis A, 23–24, 106
  hepatitis B, 29–30
  hepatitis C, 57–65
  hepatitis D, 46
  hepatitis E, 48–49
  hepatoma, 226–27
  liver tumors, 221–22
RNA test. See HCV-RNA-PCR test.

S-adenosyl-l-methionine (SAMe),
    145
Schering-Plough Corporation, 84
schistosomiasis, 161–62
sclerodactyly, 191
Scolaro, Karen and Philip, 235, 240–41,
    245, 249, 250, 264, 266
Self Healing, 97–98
self-help groups. See support groups.
serum ceruloplasmin, 14
serum glutamic oxaloacetic transaminase
    (SGOT). See aspartate
    transaminase (AST).

serum glutamic pyruvic transaminase (SGPT). *See* alanine transaminase (ALT).

serum immunoglobulin (IgM), 183

sexual transmission, of viral hepatitis, 24, 62

Shalala, Donna, 238–39

Sherlock, Sheila, 195

shortness of breath, 35, 69, 173

Sho-saiko-to, 96

sicca, 109, 180

side effects of drug therapy
   for alcohol addiction, 137–38, 139
   autoimmune hepatitis as, 108
   corticosteroids, 113, 157, 259–60
   herbal remedies, 99
   Imuran (azathioprine), 114–15
   interferon, 37–40
   for liver biopsy, 134–35
   after liver transplants, 257, 258, 259–60, 261
   pain relievers, 123–26
   Rebetron, 85–88

Silk, Adam, 120, 139–40

silymarin, 102

Sjögren's syndrome, 109, 180

skin problems, 10, 133, 191, 192

sleep disturbance, and interferon therapy, 40

spider nevi, 10, 133, 191, 201

spleen, enlarged, 27, 47, 49, 131, 134, 172, 182

Starzl, Thomas E., 236

steroid treatment, 28, 47

stools, light-colored, 27, 132

Stuart, Keith, 226, 227

support groups
   for alcoholism recovery, 137, 140–41
   for hepatitis C patients, 94

surgery
   hepatoma, 229, 232
   liver tumors, 221, 223, 224
   See also liver transplants.

symptoms
   alcoholic hepatitis, 132–33
   autoimmune hepatitis, 108–09
   cirrhosis, 68–69, 148, 151–52, 179–80
   cirrhosis (primary biliary), 177–81
   fatty liver disease, 127
   hemochromatosis, 196
   hepatic encephalopathy, 170
   hepatitis A, 26–27
   hepatitis B, 31
   hepatitis C, 66–69
   hepatitis D, 46–47
   hepatitis E, 49
   hepatoma (primary liver cancer), 214, 227
   liver cancer (metastatic), 232–33
   liver tumors (benign), 221, 222, 223
   versus signs, 10

tacrolimus, 257

tamoxifen, 231

tattooing, and hepatitis C transmission, 61

technetium sulfur colloid scan, 16, 219

telangiectasias. *See* spider nevi.

testes, shrunken, 10, 69, 152, 201

thymosin, 102–03

thymus extract, 96, 97

thyroid problems
   and autoimmune hepatitis, 109
   and interferon therapy, 36, 39–40

TIPS (transvenous intrahepatic portosystemic shunt) procedure, 166, 169

tobacco, distaste for, 27, 49

transarterial chemoembolization (TACE), 229–30

transfusion-transmitted virus (TTV), 54

transplants
   and hepatitis C transmission, 61
   and organ donation, 237–40
   See also liver transplants.

transplant team, 245–46, 250–51

transvenous/transjugular biopsy, 18–19

treatment
  alcoholic hepatitis, 136–44
  of ascites, 166–67
  autoimmune hepatitis, 112–15
  cirrhosis, 149–50
  cirrhosis (primary biliary), 158–59,
    185–92
  fatty liver disease, 129–31
  hemochromatosis, 206–08
  hepatic encephalopathy, 171
  hepatitis A, 28
  hepatitis B, 33–43
  hepatitis C, 81–103
  hepatitis D, 47–48
  hepatitis E, 49–50
  hepatoma (primary liver cancer),
    228–31, 232
  liver cancer (metastatic), 233
  liver tumors (benign), 221, 222–23,
    224–25
  variceal bleeding, 20, 114, 168–69, 210
  See also drug therapy; liver transplants.
tumor necrosis factor (TNF), 146
tumors. *See* liver tumors.
Tylenol (acetaminophen), and alcoholic
    liver disease, 123–24
tyrosinemia, 222, 226

ultrasound, 15, 77–79, 126, 153, 173,
    218
United Network for Organ Sharing
    (UNOS), 237–38, 250–51
uremia, 171
urine, dark, 27, 108, 114, 132
ursodeoxycholic acid (UDCA), 160, 182,
    185

vaccines, xii, 24–26, 30, 43, 46, 100,
    157, 234

variceal bleeding, 31, 45, 47, 69, 109,
    179, 195, 243
  and anemia, 172
  diagnosis of, 19, 20, 80, 136, 168
  risk factors for, 167–68
  treatment of, 20, 114, 136, 168–69,
    210
viral hepatitis
  acute versus chronic, 22, 31, 56–57
  blood tests, 14
  and cirrhosis, 30, 34, 68, 69, 147–48,
    156–57
  terminology, 23
  See also specific hepatitis viruses (e.g.,
    hepatitis A virus).
virologic response, 88
vitamin A, 123
vitamin C, 208
vitamin D, 189
vitamin E, 94, 160
vitamin K deficiency, 13, 75
vitamin and mineral supplements, 94,
    97, 113, 187, 189, 190

Waldenstrom, Dr., 108
water contamination, 48–49
weight gain, 78
weight loss, 31, 68, 132, 152, 179,
    187–88, 213–14
weight-reducing diet, 94
Weil, Andrew, 98
white blood count (WBC), 12, 35, 84,
    88, 133–34
Wilson's disease, xi, 14, 108, 136, 158,
    173, 242

xanthelasmas, 190

Zovirax, 261

About the Author

. . . .

DR. SANJIV CHOPRA, associate professor of medicine at Harvard Medical School and director of clinical hepatology, Department of Medicine, Beth Israel Deaconess Medical Center, Boston, Massachusetts, is also the Herrman L. Blumgart firm chief and director of the division of continuing education for the department of medicine.

Dr. Chopra has authored approximately 100 publications, including three textbooks: *Disorders of the Liver*, which has been translated into Japanese and Italian, *Pathophysiology of Gastrointestinal Diseases*, and *Gastroenterology: Problems in Primary Care*.

He is editor in chief in gastroenterology and hepatology of UpToDate, an outstanding and innovative clinical reference on CD-ROM.

Dr. Chopra has been a recipient of the George W. Thorn award, presented by the Brigham and Women's Medical House Staff. In 1991, he received the highest accolade from the graduating class of Harvard Medical School—the Excellence in Teaching award. The citation read "Outstanding Clinician, Devoted Teacher, and Mentor. We thank you for your dedication to excellence in teaching. Harvard Medical School class of 1991."

In 1995 Dr. Chopra received the Robert S. Stone award, a prestigious award given to a faculty member who is an outstanding clinician and teacher and is chosen by colleagues, house staff, and students from the Beth Israel Deaconess Medical Center, Harvard Medical School.

Dr. Chopra is widely acclaimed as a distinguished educator. He is a most sought-after speaker and has addressed medical audiences throughout the United States and several countries abroad.